A Woman's Guide to Natural Hormones

A Woman's Guide to Natural Hormones

Christine Conrad

WITH FOREWORDS BY
Leo Galland, M.D., Jesse Lynn Hanley, M.D., and
Carolyn V. Shaak, M.D., FACOG

A PERIGEE BOOK

Every effort has been made to ensure that the information contained in this book is complete and accurate. However, neither the publisher nor the author is engaged in rendering professional advice or services to the individual reader. The ideas, procedures, and suggestions contained in this book are not intended as a substitute for consulting with your physician. All matters regarding your health require medical supervision. Neither the author nor the publisher shall be liable or responsible for any loss, injury, or damage allegedly arising from any information or suggestion in this book.

A Perigee Book
Published by The Berkley Publishing Group
A division of Penguin Putnam Inc.
375 Hudson Street
New York, New York 10014

First edition: May 2000

Published simultaneously in Canada.

The Penguin Putnam Inc. World Wide Web site address is
http://www.penguinputnam.com

Library of Congress Cataloging-in-Publication Data

Conrad, Christine, 1946–
A woman's guide to natural hormones / Christine Conrad; with forewords by Leo
Galland, Jesse Lynn Hanley, and Carolyn V. Shaak.
p. cm.
Includes index.
ISBN 0-399-52581-5
1. Generative organs, Female—Diseases—Hormone therapy—
Miscellanea. 2. Hormones, Sex—Therapeutic use—Miscellanea. 3. Menopause—
Hormone therapy—Miscellanea. I. Title.

RG129.H6 C66 2000
618.1'061—dc21
99-088619

Printed in the United States of America

10   9   8   7   6   5   4   3   2   1

DEDICATED TO:

The doctors and practitioners who pioneered the use of natural hormones.

The grass-roots movement of women who insisted on better treatment for themselves.

Contents

Part One

Understanding Natural Hormones

PART TWO

Your Questions Answered

Acknowledgments

$\mathcal{M}$y deepest gratitude to: Lynette Padwa, who was a consultant on *Natural Woman, Natural Menopause*, and who worked along with me to research and write this book. She was always there with invaluable advice and editorial expertise—in addition to her warm friendship and enthusiastic support for the ideas in this book.

Leo Galland, M.D.; Jesse Lynn Hanley, M.D.; and Carolyn V. Shaak, M.D., exceptional doctors all, who are at the forefront of practicing beneficial health care for women.

Jim Strohecker, at HealthWorld Online, for his continuing support of the Natural Woman Institute.

Christine MacGenn, who has become a great friend since she worked as a researcher on *Natural Woman, Natural Menopause*.

My dearest friend, Kathy Eldon, who gives unending support to all my projects and wanted a "simplified" and easy-to-read book about hormones.

Amy Eldon, my dear adopted niece, who I hope finds this book useful for staying happy and healthy.

My exceptional agent, Jane Dystel, for her continuing care.

My lawyer, Renee Schwartz, for her always excellent advice.

Sheila Curry, my very supportive editor at Perigee, a rock in the ever-churning sea of publishing.

Joan and Gordon Page and the staff at Casa Malibu, who treated me so well when I would arrive to hole up to write at my favorite room on the ocean.

PERSONAL NOTE FROM CHRISTINE CONRAD

*G*etting information to women about natural hormones has become a personal crusade for me. My own illness and negative experiences with standard hormone replacement therapy—followed by my return to health using natural hormones—led me to write my first book, *Natural Woman, Natural Menopause* (with Dr. Marcus Laux).

Without the option of *natural* hormone therapy, I might never have recovered my own health. It was only after two years of searching—and the determination that comes from having no other choice but to continue looking—that I found a practitioner who prescribed natural hormones. In 1993, very little information or help from doctors was available. *Natural Woman, Natural Menopause* became the book that I couldn't find when I was searching for this help and information.

As with so many women, problems with hormonal balance blind-sided me. Up until my mid-forties, I had been very lucky in my health, but then a cascade of health disasters hit me: I got peritonitis and very nearly died from it; I was operated on for the bowel obstruction the peritonitis caused, then given massive doses of antibiotics, then a complete hysterectomy.

In the aftermath of the operation, I struggled for five years to recover my health. Immediately following the hysterectomy, my surgeon gave me a prescription for Premarin and said to take it the rest of my life. I remember thinking at the time, "Is this all the care I'm going to get? Isn't a hysterectomy a serious disruption of a woman's hormonal function?" At first I was able to take the Premarin (although I had some unpleasant side effects such as bloating), but then I began to have extremely serious gastrointestinal problems and could not ingest the Premarin without severe discomfort. I went from doctor to doctor, but no one could make a diagnosis. I could not eat normally and was subsisting on bland foods. I was also losing weight rapidly. Despite the severity of the malabsorption problem, no doctor would consider that my gastrointestinal distress was linked to my recent operation or the antibiotics I was given. In fact, I was given more antibiotics, which caused extreme pain and exacerbated my malabsorption and consequent weight loss. I now could not take the Premarin at all and experienced serious menopausal symptoms including severe joint pain, hot flashes, and fibromyalgia. I asked for an alternative to oral Premarin (I tried the patch but it was much too strong), but was told there wasn't one. I consulted numerous specialists, including those at a famous diagnostic clinic. The physician there told me in the first five minutes, without even looking at my charts, that all my problems were in my head. I asked the doctor to test my hormone levels, but the issue of hormone imbalance was not something this doctor considered.

Abandoned to my fate by all the practitioners I consulted, I searched on my own. When I mentioned to my internist a natural hormone cream I had heard about—which would have the benefit of being absorbed through the skin, as I could take nothing by mouth—he told me flatly that it wouldn't work and not to bother. It would be too weak. Fortunately, I ignored his advice and began using a tri-est/progesterone cream called Ostaderm—and within weeks I noticed a definite improvement. My new practitioner, Marcus Laux, a naturopath, was able to diagnose my malabsorption problems through the Great Smokies Diagnostic Laboratory. (See the Resources section on page 166.) Their tests revealed the nature of the malabsorption and the acute digestive imbalance caused by the antibiotics I had been given. Dr. Laux helped me put my gut on the road to recovery with therapies that included probiotics and plant enzymes. Then, with an added exercise and nutritional program, I began to gain my strength back.

After six months I went back to my original internist and had my hormone levels checked. He was shocked to discover I had the levels of a young menstruating female—without the periods! Later, he presented me as a case study at Cedars-Sinai Medical Center rounds, where attendees marveled that the tri-estrogen/progesterone cream had worked.

After my recovery—feeling completely healthy and transformed—I could only imagine the thousands and thousands of other women who were going through a similar ordeal. Why had information about natural hormones been so hard to find? Why had this hormone cream been dismissed out of hand when it clearly worked for me?

Many women who either have read the book I co-authored with Dr. Laux, *Natural Woman, Natural Menopause,* or have seen me on TV have reported that when they heard my story, they thought they were hearing their own. Until that time, they believed that they were alone in their misery and had nowhere to turn.

In the process of writing the book, I also realized that it was one thing to write a book on the subject, but if women didn't have access to doctors who could prescribe natural hormones for them, my job was only partly done. To that end, I founded the Natural Woman Institute, a nonprofit foundation whose primary mandate is to provide a referral service to help women find a doctor in their area and to train doctors to treat women with natural therapies. The NWI has operated a toll-free referral hotline (888-489-6626) since April 1997, averaging 250 calls a month. The Natural Woman

Institute hotline has now given doctor referrals to thousands of women.

The hotline also provides the institute with direct feedback from women all over the country. A great deal of what we hear is very dismaying. Many doctors don't want to be bothered with alternative approaches to treating menopause and hormonal imbalance issues. So many resist change, even if that change can mean a change in the well-being of their patients. One of the most common scenarios I hear is the following: A woman is given a hysterectomy and her doctor gives her a prescription for Premarin and tells her she will need to take it for the rest of her life. This woman then gains twenty-five pounds; has bloating, depression, and dry skin; and perhaps has gastrointestinal problems. She asks the doctor for an alternative to Premarin. He says there is none, or perhaps tries a few other synthetic estrogens that are no more successful, then says there is nothing more he can do. As far as this doctor is concerned, the case is closed.

But the woman continues to suffer her side effects. And she thinks she has nowhere to turn. One woman told me, "I was having trouble with the Premarin. My doctor just said that if I didn't take it, don't bother coming back when you're all bent over with osteoporosis."

Unfortunately, there is an acceptance among standard practitioners that the side effects with hormone replacement therapy (HRT) drugs are inevitable, so a woman should grin and bear it. *Side effects are not inevitable—not with natural hormones.* Today, more information is available than there was in 1993 when I first began searching, but many doctors still resist learning about natural hormones.

Can women get relief from hot flashes with the standard regime of Premarin/Provera? Certainly. But that doesn't mean it is the *best* treatment overall. Isn't it just common sense to choose a treatment that provides the same benefits but *without* the side effects and long-term risks?

Women also need to know what to do when their doctor tells them that they've reached the age where they must protect themselves against heart disease and osteoporosis, and therefore must take this pill. Many healthy women who don't want to take drugs that have side effects and risk factors are now being told to take synthetic drugs indefinitely as prevention. Again, you need to know what your options are, that there can be better, safer ways of protecting yourself.

The fact that drug companies are paying more attention to the women's market is both good news and bad news. Certainly beneficial products will be produced, but the drive for market share can press unnecessary and potentially harmful drugs on women.

Many women find the subject of hormones intimidating. And as pharmaceutical companies are now promoting natural hormone products, you need to know how to choose among them and find what's best for your particular hormonal profile. The way medicine is practiced today—the "fast-food" approach, with fifteen minutes allotted to each patient—makes it more urgent than ever that women educate themselves. I recently read with dismay a study that said that more than 60 percent of women knew nothing about the hormones estrogen and progesterone, or how hormones work in their bodies.

Fortunately, an increasing number of M.D.'s, D.O.'s (osteopaths), nurse practitioners, and other practitioners are switching from conventional HRT to the use of natural hormones. This trend is being driven in no small part by baby boomers, who are more open to the idea of using natural substances for healing. Insurance companies are beginning to recognize natural hormones as legitimate treatment that is covered by their health plans.

Still, women catch on faster than their doctors. It's estimated that only 1 percent of U.S.-trained gynecologists have any experience in prescribing and formulating natural hormone preparations. Until now, doctors have been taking their lead entirely from

pharmaceutical companies and have been fitting the woman to the
formula, not the formula to the woman.

I want to assure you that treatment with natural hormones need
not be complicated or difficult to find. *Natural hormones are now
readily available*. More information is available in books besides
this one. The compounding pharmacies that formulate natural hormones are now educating doctors and consumers via the Internet.
And growing numbers of doctors are beginning to specialize in the
midlife woman and her hormone needs. This is an important breakthrough. Until recently, a woman's hormonal issues were below the
medical field of vision. If you checked a reference book such as *Best
Doctors in America*, you would be unable to find one specialist in
this field.

Information is available on the underlying issues regarding
hormones and the politics of medicine—see the Bibliography for
suggested reading. This book gets to the heart of questions that
women have about natural hormones. A lot of unnecessary confusion has been created by the marketing of hormone drugs, and
I hope this book gives you a simple and clear explanation when a
question occurs to you. You can keep it by your desk or bedside,
or take it with you to your doctor's office. Included among the
questions are those that have been asked most often by women
calling the NWI.

FOREWORD

BY LEO GALLAND, M.D.

*I*n your quest for health, the most important thing you can do is know your own body. You are unique. There is no preset formula that will bring good health to everyone. The way you eat, the way you exercise, and the way you relax have a major impact on how you feel, but one size does not fit all.

You can learn how to understand your own individual needs by paying attention to how *well* you feel (and look), in addition to noting how specific symptoms change in response to changes in your diet, your lifestyle, or the nutritional supplements you take. If you are considering the use of hormones—for any reason—paying attention to your body is of the greatest importance. If you have already tried hormone replacement therapy and felt worse, don't be intimidated when your doctor says, "Estrogen can't cause those symptoms; they are the very symptoms that estrogen helps." You are right and the doctor is wrong, because you know your body better. Don't be discouraged, either. There are numerous alternatives to conventional hormone therapy, including nutritional supplements, herbs, and the natural hormones that are the subject of this book.

Chris Conrad has given us a guide to the use of natural hormone therapy that is practical and easy to read. As a woman who went through the system before discovering her own hormonal needs, she strongly advocates the importance of therapy that is tailor-made for each woman. She tells you how to get that therapy by managing your own health care and by working in partnership with a doctor who is willing to treat you as an individual. Increasing numbers of doctors are learning that hormonal problems cannot be treated by hormones alone. They are beginning to adopt the principles of integrated medicine, which holds that medicine works best when it helps people establish internal balance and harmony and doesn't just attempt to suppress disease.

The foundation for health and vitality at any age is a nutritious diet and a health-promoting lifestyle. Most American women derive 30 percent of their calories from nutritionally defective junk food and eat far too few vegetables. The first step in confronting the health issues raised by menopause, perimenopause, premenstrual syndrome, menstrual cramps, or irregular periods is to consume foods of high nutritional quality—including a wide variety of green, yellow, orange, and red vegetables; nuts and seeds; fruits; and seafoods—and eliminate foods containing added sugar or fat, including processed vegetable oils. The second step is to engage in regular physical exercise of moderate intensity for at least thirty minutes a day. A structured exercise program is not necessary, and your thirty minutes does not have to take place in one block of time. If your work is sedentary, altering the way you perform your everyday tasks so that you climb stairs and walk briskly for ten minutes three times a day can do wonders for your fitness level. I have seen scores of women overcome symptoms that were thought to be hormonal by simply improving their habits of diet and exercise. Nutritional supplements can also have a major impact on your symptoms.

Once the foundation for health has been laid, some women will still need natural hormone therapy to control premenstrual problems, and many will need hormone therapy to thrive after midlife. Lack of wellness, fatigue, poor sleep, loss of libido, and hot flashes are among the common symptoms that let you know you need therapies that target the changes occurring in your body as you approach menopause.

A Woman's Guide to Natural Hormones clearly explains the options available to you in hormone replacement therapy and clarifies the use of the word *natural*. Natural hormones have the same chemical structure as those made by the glands of your own body. In the case of estrogen, there are three forms: estradiol (which is the most potent), estriol, and estrone. Natural hormones are most often prescribed in a ratio that matches the ratio that usually occurs in women before menopause. Increasing numbers of doctors are beginning to recognize that individualized natural hormone therapy works better for more women than the older, conventional treatments. Natural progesterone, for example, was for many years available only from special pharmacies that compounded it themselves. Recently it has been produced by a major drug company, so it can now be prescribed by doctors through any pharmacy. This is a good sign. It tells us that the principle of individualized therapy with natural hormones is at the threshold of becoming mainstream.

Leo Galland, M.D., is director of the Foundation for Integrated Medicine (www.mdheal.org) *and the author of* Power Healing.

FOREWORD

BY JESSE LYNN HANLEY, M.D.

hen I was a young woman, menopause was portrayed as the end of the world. Now, like fifty million other women in this country, I am experiencing the awakening that menopause can bring. I have discovered that menopause is not an ending but a *beginning*. As a powerful woman elder reminded me, years ago menopause was called "the dangerous age" because at this time in her life a woman could not help but express herself and her truth, and was thus often labeled crazy. Far from being a dangerous and crazy time, I have found it to be an awakening of the wise woman within.

Unfortunately, others do not view menopause in such a positive light. Today, menopause is seen as everything from traumatic to debilitating to depressing. Deprived of ancestral guidance for this momentous transition, I began to explore cultural myths and herstories to guide me through this life change. Simultaneously, I began using natural, healthy, and safe solutions for coping with my symptoms, including herbs, exercise, good nutrition, and natural hormone creams—much of which is discussed in *A Woman's Guide to Natural Hormones*.

My recent life's work and passion has been to embrace and translate both ancient and modern safe and healthy solutions for hormonal issues for women. For over ten years in my practice at Malibu Health & Rehabilitation, I have worked to provide women with better therapies for PMS, hormonal imbalance, premenopause, menopause, and beyond. So many women have come to me with problems left untreated or mistreated, unable to tolerate the standard drugs prescribed to them. By combining centuries-old herbal wisdom with modern pharmaceutical breakthroughs, I and other practitioners have been able to provide women with solutions that are effective and safe and also gentle on the body. The scientific literature has been blossoming with new information into a woman's hormonal reality. A paradigm shift is occurring in women's medicine, as well as in women's attitudes toward taking charge of their health.

In helping the women I counsel to understand and embrace this new information, there is nothing as valuable as a great book that encompasses both the most up-to-date medical documentation and clear explanation and guidance. I loved Chris Conrad's first book, *Natural Woman, Natural Menopause*. It certainly made my work and my patients' lives easier. *A Woman's Guide to Natural Hormones* broadens the scope of the use of natural hormones to encompass women of all ages and presents it in accessible question-and-answer form. I recommend it to women of all ages as a trail guide through their passages. The clear and timely information in this book will be a welcome companion as they travel this new path.

Jesse Lynn Hanley, M.D., is medical director of Malibu Health & Rehabilitation in Malibu, California, and co-author of What Your Doctor May *Not* Tell You About Premenopause.

FOREWORD

BY CAROLYN V. SHAAK, M.D., FACOG

$\mathcal{F}$or over a decade, women interested in using natural hormones have been authoritatively told by their doctors such falsehoods as the following:

"Hormone levels can't be reliably tested."

"Natural hormones don't absorb sufficiently through the skin to protect your heart, bones, or uterus."

"Menopausal women rarely need testosterone supplements."

None of these are true. Having trained in conservative Boston (Massachusetts General Hospital, 1979–1983), I have seen firsthand the reluctance of the established medical community to venture too far afield from ingrained practices. However, I have also witnessed the serious consequences befalling women treated with conventional FDA-approved hormone therapies. I have seen the fertility ravages imposed upon DES-exposed offspring of the 1950s and have treated their cervical and vaginal cancers. I have seen 19-year-old girls paralyzed by strokes, and have seen healthy women in their thirties die from pulmonary embolism while on the overly potent birth control pills of the 1980s. Countless women suffered unnecessary uterine cancers when the conventional wisdom of the 1960s called for estrogen-only hormone replacement therapy. It is no small wonder that menopausal women, no matter how symptomatic, have serious reservations about jumping on the synthetic HRT bandwagon.

In *A Woman's Guide to Natural Hormones*, Christine Conrad provides clear and concise descriptions of the female transitions—from the onset of menses, through fertility, into menopause and beyond—as well as explanations of how natural hormones can benefit a woman at each of these stages. The questions she addresses are asked many times daily by the patients I work with at my clinic, WomenWell in Needham, Massachusetts. There is something inherently appealing to me—as a gynecologist and as a woman nearing menopause herself—about the concept of replenishing our ovarian hormones with bio-identical natural hormones. A woman using a customized natural hormone lotion will feel *every day* about the same as she used to feel before menopause. Bleeding, breast pain, weight gain, depression, and other side effects associated with oral synthetics are not generally problems for our patients. Energy, mental clarity, libido, and vaginal comfort are restored, along with the absence of hot flashes and the return of good sleep.

Too good to be true? Well, maybe, in the sense that customized natural hormone compounds are not generally available in chain drugstores. The good news is that any motivated physician and compounding pharmacy can learn to work together to create for you a customized blend of natural hormones that restores your hormonal balance safely and without side effects. Become a partner with your doctor—buy her a copy of this book—and you both will benefit from an open exchange of information. As a patient, you must be proactive. As physicians, we need only to take the time to listen, be willing to learn, and most important *believe* the symptoms we are asked to *relieve*. Enjoy a good read and share your new knowledge!

Carolyn V. Shaak, M.D., is director of WomenWell in Needham, Massachusetts, a women's health practice specializing in hormone issues.

Part One

UNDERSTANDING NATURAL HORMONES

Chapter One

WHAT ARE NATURAL HORMONES?

I had a hysterectomy at 35. . . . I have been taking Pre-marin for fifteen years and the misery keeps piling up. I am plagued with headaches, gastrointestinal problems, joint pains, you name it. . . . When I heard you speak on CNN about natural hormones, I cried. . . . There is hope for me.

(Gerry B., in a call to NWI)

*A*lthough natural hormones—also called "the naturals"—have been available to women for over fifty years in both the United States and Europe, they have not been prescribed by the majority of doctors for PMS, menopause, and hormone imbalance problems for a variety of complex reasons, mostly to do with patent laws and the way drugs are marketed.

The term *natural hormones* has come into recent common usage to differentiate these products from the synthetic and semisynthetic hormone drugs that have been most commonly prescribed to women over the past forty years. When I use it in this book I mean a hormone preparation of estrogen, progesterone, or testosterone that:

* matches your own hormones exactly—that is, it is *bio-identical*.

* is synthesized from a plant substance, either wild yam or soy.

* works in the body in the same manner as your body's own hormones.

* does not interfere with your body's own hormone production.

Only the hormones in your own body are natural in the very strictest sense. Although synthesized from plant substances in a laboratory, naturals have the same biochemical structure as your own hormones, and function in your body in the exact same way. The *natural* in *natural hormones* refers to the fact that they function in the same way as your own hormones, not to the fact that they are synthesized from a plant.

HISTORY OF NATURAL HORMONES

A breakthrough discovery in hormones was made by the chemist Russell Marker in the early 1940s. He discovered a way to replicate human hormones by synthesizing the plant substance *diosgenin,* found in abundance in the wild yam plant. Marker didn't apply for patents because he wanted to make the substance available to anyone. This proved fateful for women everywhere, because it meant that no U.S. drug company would decide to market natural hormones. Without a patent, a drug company would be unable to control the marketplace, thereby limiting potential profit.

At the time, scientific interest was focused on birth control, and Marker's discovery led to the development of a patentable synthetic version of natural progesterone—what became known as *progestin*—which was strong enough to break into a woman's menstrual cycle. The contraceptive pill was a huge success, but there was little interest in using these substances for other women's hormonal imbalance issues, such as PMS or menopause. In those years, neither PMS nor menopause were subjects addressed by the medical community.

In the 1960s, doctors began prescribing estrogen therapy for women at midlife, and millions of women began using the estrogen drug Premarin. It was promoted in the book *Feminine Forever* by Dr. Robert Wilson, a New York gynecologist, with support from the Ayerst laboratories, makers of Premarin. Dr. Wilson believed that by giving women estrogen he could save them from the ravages of what he saw as a new disease: menopause. Premarin was manufactured from horse urine (the name stands for *pre*gnant *mare*'s ur*ine*), and although it is sometimes touted as "natural" because of its animal origin, it contains estrogens that are foreign to a woman's body—it is completely natural to horses, but not to women.

At first, women were given Premarin alone, and by the 1970s approximately eight million women had been prescribed the drug. Premarin was being touted as a miracle drug that could eliminate hot flashes and night sweats and keep women "feminine forever." Then in 1977, studies done at Kaiser Permanente hospital in San Francisco showed that women on Premarin had a rate of endometrial cancer five times higher than that of non-users. Many women died from this early use of Premarin.

In order to "fix" this problem, physicians began prescribing the progestin Provera along with Premarin to protect the uterus from endometrial cancer. Progestin could balance the *unopposed* estrogen (see page 75) and protect the uterus from the proliferation of cancer cells. Provera, which uses natural progesterone as its base substance but then is altered, doesn't match your own hormones exactly and can interfere with your own progesterone production. At the time, there was little understanding of the potential negative effects of using a progestin instead of natural progesterone, and even today many physicians believe they are interchangeable.

PREMARIN/PROVERA: A FLAWED TREATMENT

The early protocols for dispensing Premarin and Provera as hormone replacement therapy (HRT) contained three fundamental scientific lapses:

1. That it makes no difference if the replacement hormone drug does not match human hormones exactly.

2. That it is not necessary to factor in the way hormones normally interact with each other when "replacing" hormones.

3. That "one size fits all," and a woman's individual hormone profile is not a significant factor.

The Premarin/Provera protocol did reduce hot flashes and night sweats, but there was also widespread dissatisfaction with the treatment. For those women who could take Premarin/Provera without side effects, it proved a benefit at least in the short term. But as many as half of all women who take Premarin/Provera stop after a year, unable to tolerate the side effects. Provera, in particular, can for a large number of women mimic PMS symptoms such as irritability, depression, water retention, and bloating. For some women, Provera proves so onerous that they choose to take Premarin alone, commonly without telling their doctors, thereby putting themselves at great risk for endometrial cancer.

There are so many side effects from Premarin/Provera because using them is like fitting a square peg in a round hole. Neither Premarin nor Provera fits exactly into *hormone receptors* in a woman's body. The poor fit manifests itself in the form of physical symptoms such as bloating, water retention, and depression. Natural hormone replacement has none of these downsides. If used appropriately, secondary side effects such as bloating or breast tenderness will not occur.

If it is important to use natural hormones instead of synthetic hormones, it is also equally important to use these hormones in balance. Any hormone replacement protocol must take into account how hormones work in the body. Giving estrogen without balancing it with progesterone not only led women to suffer side effects unnecessarily, but in the worst-case scenarios, they actually developed endometrial or breast cancer and other diseases.

These early flawed protocols left a deep scar on hormone therapy in general, as it is difficult to dissociate *any* use of hormones from the risk of cancer and from the side effects that came with the use of these two drugs. Premarin came to be synonymous with "estrogen" and Provera synonymous with "progesterone." These misrepresentations have resulted in widespread confusion and a great deal of unnecessary suffering for women.

Premarin/Provera and Synthetic Hormones: Most Common Side Effects

Bloating

Breast tenderness

Water retention

Weight gain

Agitation

Depression

Gastrointestinal problems, particularly constipation and reflux

Headaches

**Premarin/Provera and Synthetic Hormones:
Potential Long-Term Risks**

Breast cancer

Endometrial cancer

Ovarian cancer

Gallbladder disease

Liver disease

Stroke

Blood clots

For a long time a woman was given only two choices: Take the Premarin or Premarin/Provera (now also in the form of Prempro and Premphase) and suffer the side effects, or stop taking these drugs and live with the sometimes very debilitating symptoms of hormonal change.

Enter natural hormones.

NATURAL HORMONES: A BETTER SOLUTION

About twenty years ago, certain pioneer doctors and pharmacists working in the area of women's health began using what came to be known as *natural hormones*. These practitioners were looking to provide women with a safer and more side-effect–free treatment for PMS and menopausal symptoms. The basic materials were readily available. For years, major drug manufacturers such as Schering-Plough and Upjohn had been synthesizing progesterone, estrogen, and testosterone from wild yam and soy and selling it to other drug companies to use in their synthetic preparations. It became increasingly clear that the unmodified natural hormone preparations—which are FDA-approved—had the advantage of matching a woman's hormones exactly. This was not a new treatment; in Europe, natural progesterone for PMS, natural estradiol for menopause, and natural estriol for vaginal dryness and atrophy were in common usage.

Great strides were made in producing natural hormone products that were easier to use and more beneficial for women, both in treating symptoms and avoiding long-term negative effects of treatment. For example, progesterone was originally used only in suppository or injection form, but a special *micronizing* process made it available in the more practical pill form. Compounding pharmacists specializing in natural hormones developed ways to "individualize" hormone treatment and could provide it in different forms, including creams and gels, orals (pills, drops, sublinguals), and suppositories. Using hormone creams or gels, in particular, proved to have many advantages. The hormone is delivered directly to the bloodstream, bypassing the liver, thereby protecting against potential liver damage and giving an immediate systemic effect.

Today, it's estimated that over two million women are using natural hormone therapy to great satisfaction. Approximately ten thousand doctors, osteopaths, nurse practitioners, and other practitioners are prescribing this treatment nationwide. Currently, the NWI has seven thousand doctors in its database and is constantly adding new ones to the list.

Unfortunately, for a very long time there has been little incentive on the part of the drug manufacturers to change a "winning" game plan. Too often, a woman's well-being has taken a backseat to corporate profits. In addition to the unnecessary suffering of women taking Premarin/Provera, many who could benefit from hormone treatment forgo it because of their concern over side effects and long-term risks. It is only because women have begun to demand better products that the major drug companies have moved into the area of natural hormone drugs. Solvay recently received FDA approval for Prometrium, an oral natural progesterone. Wyeth-Ayerst/Columbia has Crinone, a vaginal natural progesterone preparation. More recently, Wyeth-Ayerst has begun marketing a generic natural estrogen product (estradiol).

NATURAL HORMONES AND PHYTOHORMONES

You may have heard a lot recently about plant hormones, also called *phytohormones* or *phytoestrogens*. These are not the same as the natural hormones I am discussing in this book. Plants contain substances that are similar to human hormones. When we ingest plants, they help regulate our own hormones. That is why a plant-based diet is important for both your hormonal and overall health. Extracts of phytohormones can be very beneficial for hormone balancing, and we recommend some brands. But the mandate of this book is specifically to create an understanding of natural hormones—biologically identical hormone substances synthesized from plants—as the preferred alternative to synthetic hormones.

The most important thing to understand about natural hormones is that they can provide all the benefits attributed to standard hormone replacement therapy—and even more.

The Greater Benefits of Natural Hormone Replacement

* Natural hormones match your own hormones exactly (are *bio-identical*).

* Natural hormones leave the body more quickly than synthetics, thereby not posing the same health risk.

* Natural hormones don't have the side effects of standard HRT drugs if used at the proper dosage.

* Natural hormones are natural mood enhancers; progesterone can provide this benefit, while progestin can't.

* Natural hormones can be individualized.

* Natural hormones don't interfere with your own hormone production.

* Natural hormones don't have the same long-term risks as synthetics—and are therefore much safer.

* Natural progesterone doesn't inhibit the benefits of estrogen on lowering cholesterol, as does a progestin.

* Natural progesterone will not cause you to bleed for the duration of use of HRT, as can progestin.

* Natural progesterone may protect against breast cancer.

Following is a review of all the benefits of natural hormones.

NATURAL HORMONES MATCH YOUR OWN HORMONES EXACTLY (THEY ARE BIO-IDENTICAL)

The substance you are ingesting should match the biochemical structure of your own hormones exactly. The body will recognize the substance as the same, and will process it in the same way as the hormones circulating in your body. The way molecules interact in the body is very complex and also highly specific; subtle differences in chemical structure can produce unwanted changes in the way the hormones attach to your receptors and unwanted changes in how waste is eliminated from your body, which can lead to disease.

NATURAL HORMONES LEAVE THE BODY MORE QUICKLY THAN SYNTHETICS

Enzymes in your body process your hormones. But humans do not have the enzyme to process *equilin,* the horse estrogen that constitutes half of Premarin. Levels of equilin can remain elevated for months in a woman's body because of the slow release process from fat tissue. What does this mean for the woman taking it? It means there is greater stimulation of tissue by estrogen, and this translates into a greater risk for cancer, as these horse estrogens are as much as eight times more potent than natural human estrogens in the body.

Completely synthetic estrogens are even more dangerous to you. Ethinyl estradiol is the most common form of estrogen used in birth control pills. But ethinyl estradiol is not metabolized in the liver, as is natural estradiol. It stays in the body much, much longer and may be as much as one thousand times more potent. Again, this means an overstimulation of tissue by estrogen.

NATURAL HORMONES DON'T HAVE THE SIDE EFFECTS OF SYNTHETIC HORMONES

If used appropriately, natural hormones do not have the same side effects as standard HRT. Side effects from natural hormones are tied to dose. When the dose is adjusted, most side effects will disappear. Dr. Carolyn Shaak relates the story of how when she began her gynecological practice in the 1980s, she treated patients with the standard hormone therapy that almost all gynecologists are taught in medical school. She was shocked to discover that large numbers of women suffered severely from these drugs (principally Premarin and Provera). A percentage of women could tolerate them, but a much larger percentage complained of migraines, extreme PMS-like symptoms, and excessive weight gain. All too often the side effects were worse than the original symptoms. She found it very dismaying to practice medicine this way. She then began treating her patients with natural hormones, and found that once the dose was properly adjusted through individualization, she achieved side-effect–free results and excellent patient satisfaction.

NATURAL HORMONES ARE NATURAL MOOD ENHANCERS

By restoring hormonal balance, natural hormones can relieve the anxiety and depression associated with PMS, perimenopause, and menopause symptoms. Progesterone in particular can help with sleeplessness, which in turn can relieve moodiness during the day due to lack of rest. Testosterone can promote a sense of well-being and alertness and can improve libido.

NATURAL HORMONES CAN BE INDIVIDUALIZED

Every woman has different "normal" hormone levels, and every woman's reaction to a hormone is different. This may seem self-evident, but it's an extremely important concept because drug manufacturers—and therefore doctors who prescribe their drugs—have pursued a "one size fits all" treatment. The same dose of estrogen can have decidedly different effects in different women. But fine tuning is very difficult with the synthetic hormones. With little difficulty, a compounding pharmacist can customize a natural hormone product to suit an individual woman's hormonal profile.

Natural Hormones Don't Interfere with Your Own Hormone Production

Provera, the progestin most commonly paired with Premarin, can actually lower your body's own production of progesterone. It can create a hormone imbalance, which can lead to mood swings, headaches, fluid retention, and weight gain. When given with Premarin, Provera does protect the endometrium, but the downside is considerable. Natural progesterone also protects the endometrium but without the undesirable side effects. Natural progesterone may also protect breast cells from overstimulation of estrogen, while Provera has not been shown to have a protective effect on breast cells.

Natural Hormones Don't Have Long-Term Risks and Are Much Safer Than Synthetics

One of the unfortunate facts of the highly manipulated way that estrogen has been tested for health risks is that the only estrogen that has been used for testing is Premarin! Wyeth-Ayerst not only funds studies, but provides the drug to be studied. When there has been testing of natural hormones—as in the PEPI (Postmenopausal Estrogen/Progestin Intervention) study of 1995, for example, which used both a progestin and natural progesterone in its tests—the natural hormones have shown themselves not only equal in benefits but superior to their synthetic counterparts. Clinically, natural progesterone, which has been used longest, has been proven very safe. Natural estriol, a form of estrogen, has also been used safely in Europe for over fifty years. At the very least, natural estrogen is as safe in the long term as Premarin. A noted menopause specialist, Dr. Joel Hargrove of Vanderbilt University, points out that all studies that didn't utilize natural hormones should simply be discarded as useless.

NATURAL PROGESTERONE DOES NOT INHIBIT THE BENEFITS OF ESTROGEN ON LOWERING CHOLESTEROL, AS DOES A PROGESTIN

When studying the cholesterol-lowering benefits of estrogen, the 1995 PEPI study discovered that when a progestin was added to estrogen, the potential benefit was reduced by 30 percent, whereas natural progesterone didn't diminish the effect to any significant degree.

NATURAL PROGESTERONE WILL NOT CAUSE YOU TO BLEED FOR THE DURATION OF THE USE OF HRT

For many women, one of the decided inconveniences of the Premarin/Provera regime is that they will have spotting or even periods every month even if they are past menopause. With a natural hormone regime of estrogen/progesterone, a woman may have some initial spotting that ends after a few weeks.

NATURAL PROGESTERONE MAY PROTECT AGAINST BREAST CANCER

Recent studies indicate that progesterone may protect against breast cancer. One of the most important of these studies, published in the April 1995 *Journal of Fertility and Sterility*, showed that natural progesterone inhibits estrogen's stimulation of normal breast epithelial cells. This cell stimulation can lead to breast cancer. An earlier study at Johns Hopkins in 1981 showed that breast cancer was five times higher in women with low progesterone levels than in women with higher levels.

PREMARIN/PROVERA:
AN OUTDATED THERAPY

To my mind, Premarin/Provera should be treated as outdated drugs. There is no reason to take horse estrogen when natural estrogen is available. Barry Sears, Ph.D., the scientist behind the Zone Diet, goes so far as to say, "The continued use of Premarin, which contains 50 percent of estrogens that are foreign in the human body, strikes me as one of the most ridiculous things in modern medicine."

Unfortunately, not enough physicians share this enlightened view. A woman recently told us that when she asked her female doctor about natural hormones, the doctor raised her voice and shouted, "Natural? I don't want to hear about that!" and slammed a folder of charts on her desk. A caller to the NWI said her doctor dismissed natural hormones by claiming that people are closer to a horse than a plant! As discussed earlier, the *natural* in *natural hormones* refers to the fact that the natural hormone functions identically to human hormones, not that it comes from a plant.

You may hear negative comments about natural hormones from your doctor, although this is becoming less and less the norm. It is unfortunately a common human trait to attack something you don't know about, or don't want to know about. A bad old idea can have enormous staying power, just because it's what everyone's used to. A woman can be told by a doctor who prescribes only Premarin/Provera that the naturals are not standardized, that they are not absorbed well, that they are not FDA-approved—to scare her off them and to save effort on the doctor's part. *But none of these characterizations of natural hormones are true.* The available natural products today, if obtained from competent compounding pharmacies that have well-trained staffs, are extremely reliable. They are standardized, FDA-approved substances and can be prescribed for all the indications of the standard HRT drugs.

In proper formulation, they are absorbed very well. Bear in mind that Premarin is widely acknowledged to have very poor absorption for many women.

WHO SHOULD USE NATURAL HORMONES?

For symptom relief for PMS, hormonal imbalance, and menopause, using natural hormones is the fastest, most efficacious method. Some women do very well using herbs and/or diet changes to control symptoms, but herbal remedies tend to be slow-acting and the formulas are not always reliable. If you are going to use hormone replacement, than natural hormones are in every sense a better choice. Some lucky women are just genetically capable of easily weathering hormonal storms and will not need to replenish hormones.

For long-term health benefits, such as protection against heart disease and osteoporosis, natural hormones are a much safer choice than synthetics. However, many women can do very well with a healthy plant-based diet, nutritional supplements, and a good exercise program. Other women will want to take advantage of the potential anti-aging benefits of natural hormones.

There is no question that for long-term anti-aging concerns, natural hormones can provide many benefits for skin, bone, mind, body, and overall health. In fact, the new interest in anti-aging substances arose from the initial study of female hormones. But again, this is an individual choice. We are now hearing in the media and in books of other hormones with potential benefits, such as DHEA, melatonin, human growth hormone (HGH), and pregnenolone. Read up on these substances and make your own decisions about using them. Some are discussed in the question-and-answer section. Over time, I believe that when used judiciously these substances will prove to be highly beneficial to a fit and healthy second half of life. What you don't want to do is put a synthetic product in your system, ostensibly to protect against heart disease and osteoporosis, that can then create other risks and long-term problems. There are better and safer methods.

I believe that natural hormones will become more and more the standard hormone treatment, whether through compounding pharmacies or new drugs introduced by drug companies. As doctors experience greater patient satisfaction, as the baby boom generation with their greater interest in natural substances reaches menopause, as the products themselves become more accepted and readily available—all these factors will contribute to a complete turnaround. Let's face it—until now, it has been easier to just send a woman home with a little red pill. And for many physicians, the symptoms associated with PMS, hormonal imbalance, or menopause are not their favorite subject, to say the least.

When deciding on hormone replacement therapy, it is just plain common sense to want to use the safest, gentlest, least invasive, and most risk-free form.

Chapter Two

USING NATURAL HORMONES

*T*here are basically two things you need to do to get started with natural hormones: (1) Either get your own doctor to work with you, or find another doctor; and (2) get the hormone tests you need. Testing will help establish which natural hormones you should take and then help you monitor your progress.

HOW TO WORK WITH A DOCTOR

As more doctors become knowledgeable about natural hormones, being armed with a specific battle plan will become less and less necessary, but at the present time you may encounter some resistance. I'm convinced that in as few as five years, natural hormones will become the standard treatment. For now, however, standard HRT—Premarin/Provera, in particular—is still very entrenched; it may take some patience on your part to find a doctor knowledgeable about natural hormones, particularly outside large metropolitan areas.

Although your doctor may not know about natural hormones, he or she may be one of many who have been unhappy with standard HRT. Perhaps he or she has had to deal with numerous complaints from patients and is open to learning a better way. One quick way to help convince a doctor who is on the fence is to suggest calling one of the compounding pharmacies listed in the Resources section (page 165). The compounders who specialize in naturals can provide extensive literature, technical help, reassurance, and information about proper dosing.

Or you may have a doctor who has not previously prescribed natural hormones but is open-minded enough to write the prescriptions and work with you, providing you do most of the "heavy lifting" in making the decisions about what to take, how much, and when. You can suggest to your doctor that he or she call one of the leading compounding pharmacies. In some areas of the country, this may be your only option.

If your doctor tells you he or she would like to help but is not comfortable prescribing natural hormones, that can be a legitimate position. Take the hint and look for another doctor. You want to work with someone who is knowledgeable and who understands the underlying principles of what he or she is prescribing.

Be prepared. You may very well encounter resistance from the closed-minded. You're going to get a lot of pat answers and false facts thrown at you. Some doctors will flat out tell you the naturals don't work. (You might wonder how they know they don't work if they've never tried them.) A good friend of mine told her doctor she wanted to try natural hormones and he responded, "Good grief! The next thing, it'll be coffee enemas and astrology!"

Some doctors will be very set in their ways and unwilling to listen to anything new; this is more likely to be true if they are older, but young physicians can be just as defensive. You have to realize that if they have been doling out synthetics for over thirty years and blaming complaints about side effects on emotional problems, then it stands to reason they might be resistant to hearing what you have to say.

Don't automatically assume that female doctors will be more receptive than males. They have been trained in the same medical schools and can have the same defensive attitude. A female doctor told a woman who subsequently called the NWI, "We only do Provera and hysterectomies here."

Doctors often doubt that if they substitute natural hormones they can get the same results as they do with standard HRT. But as time is proving to the millions of women now using natural hormones, they can get even *better* results.

I have noticed a tendency in women I have talked to—I felt it myself when I was ill, so I know firsthand—to be fearful that their doctor will abandon them if they go off and talk to another doctor. Perhaps it comes from a desire to be "nice," not to make waves, and to have the approval of your doctor. This is a very dangerous posture. It amounts to being willing to sabotage your own health to protect your *doctor's* feelings. It's important to be open and frank—not aggressive, not angry, just straightforward: "This is what I need. Please help me get it."

If after giving it a good try you can't work with your own doctor, call the NWI and get the lists of M.D.'s, nurse practitioners, and other doctors who are known to prescribe natural hormones.

What should you ask a new doctor? First, the obvious. Does he or she prescribe natural hormones? If so, how long has he or she been doing it? Does he or she use it as primary treatment? Many nurse practitioners—who in most states can prescribe natural hormones—will be receptive to your needs.

But even if a doctor does prescribe natural hormones, it would be unwise to go in and simply put yourself in his or her hands. The "my doctor knows everything" attitude can be dangerous to your health—especially in this time of HMOs, where doctors give as little as fifteen minutes to each patient. You must educate yourself and be an advocate for your health.

Remember, more than anything, you must be your own clinician. Pay attention to how you feel. Ultimately your body and your well-being is *your* responsibility. No one will be as attentive to your needs are you are. When you've found a medical practitioner with whom you feel comfortable, your next move will be to consider getting your hormone levels tested.

HOW TO GET THE TESTS YOU NEED

I wish there were a simple formula for hormone testing that would work for most women, but unfortunately this isn't possible. If you took a large sample of menstruating women and tested them exactly at the same time of day at the exact same point in their cycles, you would get widely disparate hormone level readings. That is because hormone levels don't have a fixed norm, as body temperature does. Hormones are complex; for some women, a slight change in levels will manifest in symptoms, while for others the same change in levels will not register at all. A 40-year-old woman may have levels that fluctuate wildly. As she gets to menopause, they may swing wider still. During menopause, a low level for one woman can be a high level for another. And in all cases, you must presuppose a doctor's ability to interpret the tests correctly. Then, too, testing is sometimes done erratically, not taking into consideration the time of day or when a woman has taken her hormone replacement—all of which can manifest themselves as widely disparate readings. To complicate matters even further, it is helpful in the beginning of a hormone replacement program to take tests at intervals of about six months, but this may prove too expensive depending on your insurance plan.

Is it possible to prescribe natural hormones without testing? Consider this: Almost all Premarin prescriptions are written without any testing whatsoever! Most gynecologists prescribe hormones for women "clinically." That is, if they have symptoms, they get a standard prescription. If the woman complains of side effects, the doctor will raise or lower the dose, ad hoc, still without reference to tested hormone levels.

Don't be overly concerned, however. If your doctor takes a good medical history and listens carefully to your recounting of symptoms, he or she can appropriately prescribe hormones without first testing your levels. Then, after a period of three or six months, if costs allow, you should get a hormone test to get a reading of your levels. If the prescription is not dealing adequately with your symptoms, the tests will be a guide to making adjustments in the protocol.

Testing can be an important tool for establishing a treatment, but understand that a test is not a judgment or a diagnosis. There is no such thing as an ideal level. Even though laboratories give indications on their reports of what a normal range is, you still have to take into account your individual profile. What you want to do is establish a *baseline test,* at which point your doctor can factor in your feedback and judge your progress during your hormone individualization program. *How you feel is the most important test of all.* It is not necessary to have absolute answers from tests to reap the benefits of therapy. Use hormone tests as a guide, not a bible.

Four types of tests are currently in use for evaluating hormone levels. The test most commonly used to determine whether a woman is in menopause—and the least informative—is the FSH/LH test. Three others offer more comprehensive measures of sex steroid hormone levels: blood, saliva, and urine tests. These three tests establish baseline levels, which give you a means of tracking progress with your hormone replenishment program. If you are over 35, you might also want to get a bone mineral density test, which measures risk or incidence of osteoporosis.

FOLLICLE-STIMULATING HORMONE (FSH) AND LUTEINIZING HORMONE (LH) TESTS

The FSH/LH blood test is the one most commonly used by physicians to determine whether a woman is in menopause. It is a rather simplistic measure as it doesn't test the levels of estrogen, progesterone, testosterone, and other sex steroid hormones. It tests for levels of follicle-stimulating hormone (FSH) and luteinizing hormone (LH). These two hormones, secreted by the brain, play a part in the rise and fall of estrogen and progesterone during your menstrual cycle. Measuring their levels—essentially how hard these secondary hormones have to work to regulate your cycle—can provide an indicator of whether you have stopped ovulating. But these tests can be very inaccurate, and can give conflicting results depending on the time of month they are administered. According to Dr. Carolyn Shaak, using the FSH test alone can be very misleading, as it is not a measurement of hormonal levels so much as an indicator of how loudly the brain must "scream" at the ovary to get it to work. FSH can be high, but the ovary can respond well with normal estradiol (E2) levels. A woman can test positive for menopause one week, at which time her doctor prescribes HRT drugs, but two weeks later a further test may indicate she is not menopausal! The prescription for estrogen may in fact exacerbate her present symptoms.

BLOOD SERUM PANELS

Blood serum hormone levels are extensively used to monitor hormone response during in vitro fertilization cycles, and they are likewise a useful tool if used correctly in monitoring hormone replacement therapy. If a woman is using a long-acting supplement, such as a transdermal cream applied to fatty areas (hips/abdomen/thighs), blood levels will be relatively stable over all hours of the day and hormone testing can occur at any time. However, if oral preparations (such as Prometrium and Estrace) are used, levels will fluctuate dramatically according to the time of blood testing relative to the ingestion of the pills. If you are not using hormone supplements and are still having occasional periods, your blood levels may vary dramatically according to where you are in your cycle. Your physician needs to be aware of your cycle day and any hormonal supplements you are using to factor this into his or her interpretation of your values. "Free" hormone levels (the biologically active component in your blood) are necessary when evaluating testosterone and thyroid levels. To ensure that patients absorb transdermal creams, and to evaluate whether the ratios of progesterone, estrogen, and testosterone are correct in these creams, blood hormone levels are an essential tool for your practitioner.

SALIVA TESTING

This newer form of hormone testing has recently become available to the general public. With blood tests you get a reading of the total hormone content of your blood for both *bound* hormones—which are bound by protein and essentially held in abeyance for future use—and *free* hormones, which are actively seeking receptor sites. The level of free hormones in the blood is about 2 percent of total content. Free hormones enter the saliva through the cells of the salivary glands and therefore you can get a reading of the free hormones that are circulating in your body and actively interacting with your hormone receptors. Proponents of saliva testing point out that with blood tests you can only estimate the level of, say, free estrogen; a saliva reading is a more accurate indicator.

This test is certainly more user-friendly in that it can be done at home and there are no needles! At this time doctors commonly speak in a language of "blood levels"; for many M.D.'s, translation into saliva levels is uncomfortable and may limit their ability to accurately adjust your medication. Saliva levels can be almost effortlessly collected over a time period of a few weeks, and can help paint a hormonal portrait of a woman who is still menstruating irregularly. As more data is amassed and more doctors become familiar and comfortable with it, saliva testing will undoubtedly gain wide acceptance. (See the Resources section, page 165).

24-HOUR URINE TESTING

Jonathan Wright, M.D., a leading specialist in natural hormones, prefers using a 24-hour urine test. This is because hormones are secreted in "pulses," and a single drawing of blood or saliva collection may not provide a representative sample. But this test is obviously not the most user-friendly or desirable method, and most doctors are unfamiliar with it.

As more doctors begin to specialize in hormone issues they will necessarily become more familiar with testing procedures. If your own doctor is unwilling to administer hormone tests, call the NWI for a referral in your area.

BONE TESTING

In addition to testing your hormone levels, you will want to find out how your bones are doing in terms of both their overall density and the rate of bone loss. After 35, a woman begins to lose bone at an accelerated rate. These tests will also establish a baseline and be the foundation of a program to increase your bone strength and arrest any bone loss.

There are several methods of assessing the status of your bone density. *Dual-energy X-ray absorptiometry (DEXA)* measures your bone density at a single point in time. It measures the density of the bones in your spine, forearm, and hip and compares them with that of a woman at peak bone mass (age 35). If you are in your late thirties or older, a normal result would be less than one standard deviation below peak bone mass. The higher the number of standard deviations, the larger the deviation between your bone mass and peak bone mass. Osteoporosis occurs at a standard deviation of 2.5 or higher. If your doctor says you are at risk for osteoporosis, it means your deviation is somewhere between 1 and 2.5 (ask the exact number if you're curious).

Some less expensive versions of this test are available in chain drug stores and other locations; these tests measure bone density at the heel or wrist.

Ultrasonographic bone densitometry uses sound waves to

measure bone mineral density (BMD). Recently approved by the FDA, this test is proving to be a popular tool as it is quick, painless and non-invasive. It measures the transmission of high-frequency sound waves through your heel bone. Unlike DEXA, you are not exposed to any level of X-ray radiation.

Both of the preceding tests are good tools for determining the present condition of your bones and whether you are at risk for osteoporosis. But for a more complete picture of the health of your bones, you need to combine either test with a urine test, *deoxy-pyridinoline (Dpd)* (also called *Pyrilinks-D*), which gives you a reading of how quickly you are *losing* bone. Dpd is an important marker of bone breakdown. (A similar test called NTx, also reads bone breakdown.) If you are losing bone rapidly, you are definitely a candidate for hormone replenishment. Ideal collection time is your first or second urination of the day. If you are using a calcium supplement with bone meal, be sure you have not taken any supplement for 48 hours prior to taking this test.

By combining information from both the DEXA (or ultrasonic) and Dpd tests, your doctor can get a complete picture of the health of your bones and predict whether you are a candidate for fractures in the future. Once you have begun hormone replenishment, you can take the Dpd test at specified intervals to assess the progress of your therapy.

One caveat about osteoporosis tests. As valuable as they can be, they can also be an excuse to put women on osteoporosis drugs they can do without. You may show some bone loss on your test that can be corrected with a good exercise program (that includes weight-bearing activities as well as strength training) and diet (including foods high in calcium), and then perhaps hormone replenishment—without adding drugs that have side effects and long-term risk factors.

Chapter Three

DIET, SUPPLEMENTS, AND EXERCISE — KEYS TO HORMONAL HEALTH

DIET

Using natural hormones at any time—whether for PMS, hormonal imbalance, or menopause—should never be a substitute for taking care of your overall health. In fact, they should not be seen as separate issues. You should be supporting your hormones nutritionally all through your life. The healthier you are, the better your hormones balance and communicate with one another. If you're taking natural hormones but continuing a bad diet, you are working against your health. Every day, new information arrives that tells us about the interaction of food and the hormones in your body.

You may have heard a lot recently about the benefits of soy in a diet. Soy contains beneficial substances called *phytohormones*, which interact with and help regulate your own hormones, raising or lowering your hormone levels as needed. Recent research on the Asian diet brought attention to the fact that Asian women have a lower incidence of breast cancer and fewer menopausal problems than Western women. When these Asian women changed to a Western diet, they began to experience more illness and more menopausal symptoms.

The all-too-common American diet of hamburgers, fries, other fast foods, lots of sugar-loaded desserts, coffee all day long, and foods that in general have little nutritional value or are loaded with preservatives is not only bad for your overall health but is also bad for your hormonal health. If you have a particularly high-fat diet, you are actually increasing your estrogen levels and keeping estrogens circulating in your body instead of eliminating them as quickly as is desirable. A high-fiber diet can help eliminate estrogens quickly and keep them from recirculating. Because the Japanese diet is low in fat and high in fiber, Japanese women have half the levels of circulating estrogen compared to those of American women, and a much lower breast cancer rate.

Certain foods can increase symptoms of hormonal imbalance. If you drink too much coffee and eat too many spicy foods around the time of your period, you can increase the intensity of symptoms of PMS; these same foods can increase the intensity of hot flashes during menopause.

These are just a few examples of how diet and hormones interact. All too often a women gets an alarm signal in the form of hormone problems to tell her she is nutritionally deficient.

You've probably been hearing a lot lately about herbal medicine. It's now known that traditional herbs used by women for so-called female complaints contain phytohormones, which interact with and regulate human hormones. Herbs such as black cohosh, dong quai, vitex agnus-castus, and wild yam, to name a few, have been helping woman with menstruation, childbirth, and menopause for as long as five thousand years.

Dr. Leo Galland reports success using fish oils to reduce menstrual cramps and breast pain. He says that evening primrose oil and flaxseed oil can also be helpful for premenstrual syndrome. These oils can boost your body's ability to make or respond to estrogen and progesterone. You are especially likely to need supplements of these oils if you are troubled by dry skin and hair; soft, fraying, or brittle nails; or a recent onset of hot flashes. Vitamin E and selenium help your body utilize the oils more effectively and may also help premenstrual, menstrual, and early menopausal symptoms. Supplements of calcium or magnesium can be very helpful, especially if you are troubled by insomnia, anxiety, irritability, muscle tension and spasm, heart palpitations, or migraine headaches. These minerals have the added advantage of helping to ward off osteoporosis.

For some women, simple changes of diet, or using herbs, with the addition of an exercise regime can help stabilize their hormones. If that's all it takes for you—meaning your symptoms have disappeared—you may not need to use natural hormones.

You can practice preventive hormonal medicine by improving your diet. Help your female friends and relatives understand that eating right is your best defense against hormonal imbalance problems. Eat a healthy diet and you may be one of those women who avoid PMS or sail through menopause without symptoms. This same good diet—particularly a diet that is heavily skewed to vegetables and fruits—can protect you against breast cancer and other cancers.

Many good books spell out in greater detail how to follow a diet that is hormonally beneficial. (See the Bibliography, page 197, for further listings.) Here's a simple list of changes you can make that will greatly improve your health and well-being.

Dietary Changes You Can Make Immediately

* Eliminate refined sugar or artificial sweeteners; replace them with honey or Sucanat (natural sugar cane).

* Drink six to eight glasses a day of pure water—free of chlorine and fluoride.

* Avoid diet sodas and soft drinks, which have a high phosphorus content and leach minerals from your bones.

* Reduce or eliminate coffee consumption. If you do

drink coffee, make it organic, but substitute herbal, green, or black tea wherever possible.

* Reduce alcohol consumption.

* Try to eat organically grown, whole foods. They are more readily available and affordable today than they have been in the past.

* Avoid processed food and artificial flavorings, colorings, or preservatives.

* Reduce animal fat consumption. Eat red meat sparingly, favoring poultry and fish whenever possible. In fact, increase consumption of fish, particularly salmon and tuna, which contain beneficial essential fatty acids (EFAs) your body doesn't make itself.

* Avoid synthetic drugs wherever possible. Don't automatically use antacids, painkillers, and tranquilizers.

* Eliminate tobacco.

SUPPLEMENTS

In addition to maintaining a healthy diet, pay attention to your digestion. You can be eating all the right foods, but if your digestion is poor you will not be absorbing nutrients properly—or, for that matter, providing the right environment for the way hormones circulate and are then eliminated from your body. The relative health and balance of your intestines is vital to both your general health and how you use any natural hormones you take. Plant digestive enzymes help your system digest and absorb the nutrients in your food. *Probiotics*—"good" bacteria—are supplements that help maintain the balance of your intestinal flora and prevent the proliferation of "bad" bacteria, which can compromise both your overall and hormonal health.

Also consider adding other nutritional supplements to your diet. Let's face it—our present-day environment is extremely taxing. The general stress of daily living, pollutants from the environment, and foods that are nutritionally deficient and contain pesticides and chemicals put extra pressure on our bodies, particularly our immune systems. In addition to choosing a healthy diet, you can further protect yourself with vitamin, mineral, and nutritional supplements.

An extensive survey of what is available to you is outside the scope of this book, but many other books can give you more detailed information. (See the Bibliography.) Also consider getting a test to determine what vitamin deficiencies you might have. An excellent test is available from SpectraCell Laboratories. (See Resources.) You will need a doctor's prescription.

Supplements You Can Add to Your Daily Regimen

∗ *A broad-spectrum multivitamin and mineral supplement.* Refined foods can be very low in mineral content. It is best to use a multivitamin complex, not high doses of single vitamins. Choose a product that is specifically geared to a woman's hormonal balance and to the support of her bones. The "just take calcium" dictum is less than worthless; you need a supplement that also includes magnesium, boron, and zinc, among other minerals, which help metabolize calcium to prevent osteoporosis.

∗ *An antioxidant formula.* These formulations include the vitamin C, vitamin E, beta-carotene, and selenium. There are many good products on the market, including Prevail's Antioxidant Formula and Enzymatic Therapy's Doctor's Choice Antioxidant. Antioxidants protect against so-called *free radical* damage in the body, which is directly related to most diseases in your body, and can help support your immune system and prevent osteoporosis. They also protect against outside pollutants, xenoestrogens, and nutritional deficits. (See "Recommended Products" in the Resources section.)

* *Essential fatty acids (EFAs)*. More and more attention is being paid to the benefits of these nutrients, which are particularly found in cold-water fish such as tuna and salmon, and in seed oils. They can help normalize your hormones, protect your arteries, and maintain ideal weight. You will find good products in health food stores.

* *"Green" foods*. Chlorella, spirulina, wheat barley, and alfalfa grasses are examples of this category of nutritional supplement. Chlorella and spirulina are wonderful sources of vegetable protein to supplement a diet deficient in them. They contain a wealth of concentrated digestible proteins, amino acids, and vitamins and minerals. Health benefits include reducing cholesterol levels, increasing hemoglobin levels, improving digestion, and eliminating dangerous toxins from your body.

* *Digestive enzyme supplements*. These supplements help the body break down food into nutrients that can be used more effectively. So many factors inhibit our digestion—aging, stress, drugs, and environmental factors, among others. Enzyme supplements also can help ensure you're getting the full benefit of natural hormones.

* *Probiotics*. These supplements contain species of healthy intestinal flora such as *acidophilus* and *bifidus* to support your digestive tract.

EXERCISE

The benefits of exercise extend far beyond just simple cosmetic changes in your appearance. For your general health, exercise can lower your blood pressure, sharpen your memory, protect against heart disease, decrease your risk of breast cancer by 50 percent, increase your bone density and strength, increase blood circulation, tone and smooth your skin, and give you energy, not to mention keeping you looking younger and more vital. It also has important benefits for hormonal balance, although here the key is regular but moderate exercise. Too much strenuous exercise can interfere with ovulation, for example, whereas little or no exercise slows down the effectiveness of your metabolism, which in turn can affect how you process both nutrients and your hormones.

Try to do some exercise daily, even if it means just walking briskly twenty minutes a day. It is your best defense against all aspects of aging. I recommend strength (or weight) training as one of the best forms of exercise for women. In terms of its general health benefits, the amount of time you need doing it, how quickly you will begin to see results, and how reliable it is in giving you results, it beats all other forms, such as swimming and cycling, by a mile. It is the only form of exercise that can actually reverse loss of bone density.

Weight training will increase flexibility, increase endurance, reduce body fat, add lean muscle tissue, increase energy and confidence, increase balance and tensile strength, and improve your body composition. It is a particularly good form of exercise if you're non-athletic. Anyone can do it—even 90-year-olds. You just have to start at your own level, and gradually increase weight at your own pace. No matter what form of exercise you choose, it is important to do something!

Exercise Changes You Can Make Immediately

* Sign up for a strength training program at your local gym. Take a friend to keep you company. Invest in a personal trainer for a least a few sessions. It is important to know the correct way to use machines and/or weights. Most gyms have trainers on staff.

* Do some stretching exercises every day. Stretching is extremely important in maintaining a youthful flexibility, reducing stress, extending your range of motion, and improving your joints. Even little stretches throughout the day will help. Always do some arm and shoulder stretches every twenty minutes while at the computer or sitting in one position for a length of time.

* At the very least, walk briskly for a minimum of twenty minutes a day. If you can't always do that, add in extra physical movement—for example, if you can take the stairs instead of the elevator, do it.

The combination of a healthy diet, supplements to augment that diet, and exercise that keeps you moving and strong will go a long way to make you feel good and look good as well as keeping you healthy.

Chapter Four

FINDING YOUR HORMONAL PROFILE

$\mathcal{F}$rom the time she begins menstruating, a woman's overall well-being will be directly affected by the balance of the hormones that govern her monthly cycles. Even after your monthly cycles begin to wind down and then end, your health will still be affected by the balance of hormones in your body. Finding yourself in these profiles will help you get a good handle on how to resolve any "female problems" safely and quickly as they come along, without resorting to more drastic measures. But remember, we are all unique, with our own genetic predisposition and life situations, and what describes you may not necessarily apply to another woman. Pay attention to yourself. You are the best custodian of your own health. The more you understand how your body works, the more likely you are to progress easily and healthfully through these transitions.

PMS (PREMENSTRUAL SYNDROME) AND HORMONAL IMBALANCE

PMS

A young woman suffering with PMS might be shocked to discover that PMS was not officially recognized as a real syndrome until the 1970s. When it comes to hormones, science has been a very slow learner. Her mother is likely of a generation who went to the doctor with the same symptoms only to be told it was all in her head, then given a prescription for tranquilizers! This may be very hard to believe now, but it speaks to how primitive the understanding of the workings of a woman's body has been and the basic neglect relating to understanding the hormonal system. In fact, the first U.S. study that linked PMS, estrogen, and progesterone was published in 1997 in the *New England Journal of Medicine*.

Many doctors still insist that hormone balance has nothing to do with PMS; that the syndrome is purely psychological. But any woman who has had PMS can tell you the symptoms are very real indeed. However, no two women will experience PMS the same way. Women differ greatly in the way they respond to monthly cycles:

* Some women are more sensitive than others to hormonal fluctuations.

* Some women have difficult periods all their lives (a small percentage).

* Some have mild symptoms that vary from month to month (the largest percentage).

* Some have mild symptoms until their thirties, which then become increasingly severe as they head toward menopause (the most common scenario). In fact, heavy bleeding and cramping are the common menstrual symptoms of perimenopause and can often lead to an unnecessary hysterectomy.

* Some have anovulatory (lack of ovulation) cycles, which, though unrecognized, can cause menstrual distress such as swollen breasts, cramps, and mood swings.

To all the myriad variations on a woman's response to the fluctuations of hormones in her system, it's also necessary to add the factors that can exacerbate symptoms: improper diet, lack of exercise, stress, and emotional issues.

PMS is described as a *syndrome*, meaning it encompasses a very long list of possible symptoms.

The Most Common Symptoms of PMS

* cramping

* bloating

* water retention

* breast tenderness

* breast enlargement

* back pain

* irritability

* headaches

* anxiety

* mood swings

* depression

Beginning sometime within the two weeks before your period, you can begin having symptoms—one or any combination of those listed here—that usually increase in intensity until menstruation begins or a few days into menstruation, and then finally subside.

But just because PMS is a very common complaint doesn't mean it is an *inevitable* complaint. A great deal can be done to mitigate the symptoms of PMS. Treatment with progesterone is at the top of the list.

The use of progesterone for PMS symptoms was introduced

by an English physician, Dr. Katherina Dalton, in the 1940s. She was in the forefront of getting PMS to be recognized as a real syndrome, not simply something "in your head," then treating the symptoms with progesterone. For over forty years, she used progesterone to control symptoms of PMS with excellent results.

Following Dr. Dalton's lead, certain pioneering U.S. compounding pharmacies, such as Madison Pharmacy, began compounding progesterone in suppository form in this country in the 1980s. More recently, Dr. Joel Hargrove of Vanderbilt University Medical Center, a recognized expert in natural hormones, has done studies that have demonstrated a 90 percent success rate treating PMS with oral progesterone.

I used progesterone suppositories for PMS in the early 1980s, when it was a relatively unknown treatment in this country. My gynecologist gave me a prescription for them, saying with a shrug, "Try them, maybe you'll get some relief." I think back now with amusement at how skeptical and naive I was, thinking, "Oh my God, I'm taking *hormones!* I'm way too young!" But I did use them, and they were *extremely* effective, and I was very grateful. I realize I was like so many women who didn't have the faintest idea how my periods worked and what could cause PMS. There is so much more information available now; you don't have to be as naive as I was.

It has become common recently to treat PMS with antidepressants such as Prozac, and the manufacturers of these products have been heavily promoting this usage. There is evidence of some relief from symptoms—serotonin levels are linked to estrogen levels, and antidepressants raise serotonin levels—but there is no reason to resort to such a drastic measure when progesterone works even better.

Women with very severe PMS may need to take progesterone monthly, and perhaps continuously through the years; others will find that they can use it as needed in months when they are particularly symptomatic.

Although progesterone can be helpful to many women, you must also work on other fronts to deal with symptoms. To repeat, every woman is different. Her life circumstances are different, her basic genetic makeup is different, her diet is different. For some women, sometimes simply eliminating coffee in the two weeks before a period can make a huge difference in how she feels. Then, by adding other dietary changes, exercise, and nutritional supplements, she can go a long way toward wiping out monthly misery.

PMS Action Plan

* Talk to your doctor about progesterone. A transdermal cream or suppository can be made up for you by a compounding pharmacist. I recommend you try the cream or suppository form first. If they don't work, you can try oral micronized progesterone.

* Over-the-counter products such as Pro-Gest, Kokoro Balance Cream, and other progesterone cream products can also be very effective. Follow instructions on the packaging for PMS.

* A good multivitamin and mineral supplement can help a great deal. Check a health food store for supplements geared for women.

* Eliminate caffeine altogether or drastically reduce consumption, especially during the two weeks before your period.

* Eliminate refined sugar and carbohydrates.

* Avoid birth control pills.

* Start an exercise program. Walking is very important. But if you're a woman who exercises extensively, don't go to extremes just before your period.

* Remifemin, an herbal product containing the phytoestrogen black cohosh, can help with hormonal balance and is very effective for PMS.

PMS is not "in your head." It is a very real syndrome with very real symptoms. The good news is that there are effective strategies and treatments that can reduce or eliminate your PMS symptoms.

HORMONAL IMBALANCE

By the time a woman reaches her thirties, a number of problems can manifest themselves. They are not necessarily life-threatening; they are not diseases per se. They are, as they have been euphemistically called, "female problems."

The list includes the following:

* endometriosis (excess growth of endometrial tissue, which causes severe pain and cramping before and during periods)

* enlarged uterus (causes menstrual discomfort)

* uterine fibroids (growths on the uterus)

* fibrocystic breasts (lumpy and painful breasts)

* anovulatory cycles (lack of ovulation)

* excessive bleeding

* irregular bleeding

It is beyond the scope of this book to go into detail on each of these disorders and their possible treatments, but what I want to concentrate on here is how understanding these problems as fundamentally related to hormone imbalance, and using natural hormones to restore balance, can mitigate them significantly or put them out of your life entirely. Every single one of these "female problems" can be related back to an imbalance between your estrogen and progesterone.

But first, understanding a few fundamental principles of your monthly menstrual cycle will go a long way to helping you understand how these problems can come about.

FIGURE 1

Hormone Levels of the Menstrual Cycle

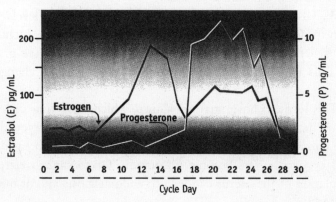

THE MONTHLY ESTROGEN/PROGESTERONE SEESAW

Every month in a menstruating woman, estrogen and progesterone rise and fall in an essentially seesaw pattern. (See Figure 1.)

In the first part of your cycle, following the end of menstruation, estrogen levels rise, stimulating the lining of your uterus in preparation for a possible pregnancy. At this time, your progesterone levels remain low.

In the middle of your cycle, there is a surge of estrogen just before an egg is released from your ovary.

Now it's progesterone's turn. After ovulation, there is a surge of progesterone, to prepare your uterus for the implanting of a fertilized egg.

If the egg becomes fertilized, your progesterone remains high and will stay that way to maintain the lining of the uterus during your pregnancy. If there is no fertilization of the egg, your progesterone falls back down to a low level.

Up/down, up/down—this monthly seesaw continues through your fertile years.

In your twenties, the ratios maintained by estrogen and progesterone to each other normally remain steady, which shows up as regular and uneventful periods.

As you get into your thirties, your progesterone levels may begin to decrease due to a number of different factors, including diet, genetics, stress, and exposure to xenoestrogens (see p. 82), and thus your *ratio* of estrogen to progesterone may change as well.

This leads to hormonal imbalance, which, over time can lead to the "female problems" listed here. For example, if you don't have enough progesterone to balance estrogen, your breasts can swell or, worse yet, become fibrocystic. Or too much estrogen stimulation of the uterus can lead to endometriosis and/or uterine fibroids.

Because gynecologists tend to treat these problems as distinct and unrelated to hormone imbalance, they are approached piecemeal and are frequently worsened by the wrong treatment. To "attack" the problem, women are usually given progestins (such as Provera) or birth control pills (synthetic estrogen and/or synthetic progesterone versions). While some temporary relief can be gained from these drugs, in the long run they can worsen the problem. When there is no resolution to the problem, more radical surgery is recommended—first a D&C (dilation and curettage) for heavy bleeding, where the lining for the uterus is scraped away to then grow anew, and then the most radical, a hysterectomy. This unfortunate scenario can keep a woman in a never-ending cycle of returning to the doctor's office for chronic problems, continuing discomfort, and if perhaps not shutting down her life altogether, giving her a significantly diminished existence.

Your thirties and forties become a high danger zone for intervention with synthetic drugs and surgery. A much better first line of defense is using a natural progesterone cream during the monthly cycle for balance and to eliminate estrogen dominance, that is, excessive levels of estrogen relative to progesterone. If this doesn't work, other approaches can be considered.

Major drug manufacturers are now beginning to catch on to the benefits of natural progesterone to restoring hormone balance and normal functioning of the menstrual cycles. Crinone, produced by Wyeth-Ayerst, is a natural progesterone gel recently approved by the FDA for anovulation. Although the product itself is a messy blue gel that many women don't like, it is a step in the right direction in terms of its basic approach and the science behind it—that is, using a natural progesterone instead of a synthetic progestin. Using a progestin can be effective to some degree, but it can come with significant side effects.

Surprisingly, the number of U.S. women who actually stop having periods before age 40 is in the millions. The standard treatment for these women is either the progestin Provera or a progestin-based birth control pill. Although a progestin can alleviate symptoms, progesterone is preferable for all the reasons given earlier. In addition, Dr. Jesse Lynn Hanley reports many more women in her practice who are having severe menstrual problems, such as heavy bleeding and clotting, than in previous years. A number of researchers and doctors have pointed to environmental and dietary factors adversely affecting individual hormone levels, which may be behind this phenomenon. To combat this problem, a woman may need to add a regular regimen of vitamins and minerals and nutritional supplements.

BREAST CANCER SURVIVORS

The underlying cause of breast cancer can also be viewed as a hormonal imbalance problem (so-called estrogen-sensitive breast cancer), but obviously here we are dealing with a serious disease, not just monthly discomfort.

If you're taking tamoxifen, you may be experiencing menopausal symptoms such as hot flashes and night sweats. Many doctors prescribe natural progesterone to these women. You can also try Remifemin to help with hormonal balance. It is considered safe for breast cancer survivors.

The next step may be the use of estriol. See the question-and-answer sections in Chapters 5 through 12 for a complete description of the potential benefits of estriol. If you do decide to use estriol, always do so in conjunction with progesterone.

Hormonal Imbalance Action Plan

* Your first line of defense for any hormonal balance problem is to look to your nutrition, stress levels, and exercise habits (or lack of them). Follow the diet and exercise prescriptions in Chapter 3 and the general guideline relating to PMS.

* Consider using natural progesterone.

* See Chapter 7 for specific recommendation for endometriosis and fibrocystic breasts.

PERIMENOPAUSE

For a woman, perimenopause invariably comes too soon. Although the root *peri-* literally means "surround," perimenopause generally refers to the time when a woman is still menstruating, albeit more erratically, and when her body begins to show the signs and symptoms of hormonal shifting and reduced production. Perimenopause can occur over a few years or over as many as ten, and most commonly begins in the mid-forties. It is very much like menopause without the actual cessation of monthly periods.

For many women this is by far the most challenging time because the denial factor can be so powerfully active. Each sign of change in a woman's body can activate her fear of losing her position of "youth" in society. Just admitting that change is happening can be a difficult hurdle. By the time a woman actually stops menstruating, she is often more mentally prepared to move into the next stage of life than she was when perimenopause began.

To compound the problem, a woman may receive little help or sympathy from her doctor. Women in perimenopause are the forgotten women; if the menopausal woman is often neglected, then the perimenopausal woman is doubly so. Doctors themselves typically have little information about this phase and frequently misdiagnose and/or mistreat the symptoms. It can be a time when bad dietary and exercise habits come home to roost and a woman's body sends signals that it can no longer tolerate them.

Take heart: Every symptom can be dealt with and you can actually feel better than you did in your thirties. True, we can't turn back the clock, but the woman who pays attention, begins to make some changes, and avails herself of the appropriate remedies, will be rewarded with renewed vigor and prepared to make the second part of life the best part of life.

Signs of Perimenopause

* Your periods begin to change.

* You experience night sweats.

* You experience hot flashes.

* You have trouble sleeping.

* You experience depression—and not just around your period, as before.

* You begin gaining weight; you're not metabolizing fats and carbohydrates as you once did.

* Your skin is changing, losing its elasticity.

* You notice a drop in libido and the loss of vaginal lubrication.

* Sometimes you can't concentrate and are forgetful.

These symptoms are also the symptoms of menopause. But for many women, symptoms begin *before* they stop menstruating and can continue for several years. "The change" happens gradually over a number of years; the actual cessation of bleeding is a nonevent.

It is important to understand that changes in your cycle don't necessarily signal that something is wrong. A woman can panic and think the changes in her period are a sign of abnormality, without realizing that she's just entering a phase of hormonal shifting. What is happening is that hormone levels are gradually dropping below a point necessary to create a menstrual cycle. If your cycle has been like clockwork every twenty-eight days, you may now find you are getting your period every three weeks, or every twenty-five to twenty-six days. The degree of cramping may increase. Also, your flow may change from "normal" to a less heavy flow that lasts only three days. Another possible scenario is a longer cycle, say every thirty-five to forty days, or a cycle that skips a month every so often. Every woman responds differently to this time when hormone production begins tapering off.

WHAT CAN YOU DO?

You can mitigate all of the symptoms and put yourself on the road to an even better state of health for the future. Unfortunately, too many women are told, "Just live with it." Others are given the wrong treatment. Many women in perimenopause are prescribed estrogen during a time when their estrogen levels are fluctuating dramatically. Adding estrogen frequently exacerbates the problem or gives a woman PMS-like symptoms, such as mood swings, headaches, and bloating. (These women do well using progesterone alone to relieve symptoms.) Worse still, some doctors prescribe antidepressants to relieve depression caused by hormone imbalance. Severe menstrual changes often lead to prescription of a hysterectomy during this time, which can create even greater problems.

Perimenopause Action Plan

* First, get baseline hormone levels checked by following the suggestions in Chapter 2.

* Examine your diet using the guidelines in Chapter 3 and begin to make changes that can mitigate symptoms, such as eliminating or reducing coffee, alcohol, and spicy foods.

* Begin an exercise program immediately. Exercise can both help prevent bone loss *and* reduce or eliminate perimenopausal symptoms.

* Look at all the stress factors in your life and try to eliminate as many as you can. Stress can exacerbate symptoms.

* Begin taking vitamin, mineral, and herbal supplements as recommended in Chapter 3.

* If your hormone levels warrant it, among the most effective treatments to ameliorate symptoms are the herbal supplement Remifemin, progesterone cream, and if necessary, a combination of estrogen and progesterone. An over-the-counter progesterone cream may be sufficient for you if your body responds quickly to it and your symptoms are mild. Otherwise, you will need a progesterone preparation with a larger amount of progesterone prescribed by your physician.

* Take note about estrogen replacement: It can frequently exacerbate a problem at a time when your estrogen levels are fluctuating. Progesterone alone can deal with symptoms during this time.

SURGICAL MENOPAUSE

The number of women who have hysterectomies and are in surgical menopause is, sadly, vastly too large. It's been estimated that as many as 80 percent of hysterectomies are unnecessary. The average age of a woman in this category is 35, and by age 60 nearly half of American women have been hysterectomized. What should only be an extreme choice is done too often without regard to consequences. For far too long, millions of women have been silent sufferers.

I am particularly dismayed by the callers to the NWI who had hysterectomies in their thirties or even their twenties, and who then have suffered from negative symptoms for years and even decades afterward. Besides being deprived of their childbearing capabilities, they have lived with chronic ill health that has robbed them of vitality and sexuality—literally taking away precious years of their youth.

Beware of practitioners who think of a hysterectomy as a routine procedure. It may be routine for them, but *you* have to live with its consequences. One of the most common reasons for a hysterectomy is painful uterine fibroids. If using natural progesterone doesn't shrink your fibroids, you should look into a new procedure called a uterine artery embolization, which has shown promise in offering relief without resorting to the removal of the uterus. Once you've had a hysterectomy—frequently with the promise that it will resolve whatever problems you are having—there are serious shortfalls in dealing with your well-being after the operation. Generally, women are sent home with a prescription for Premarin and told to take it for the rest of their lives.

Those responsible for the operation tend to minimize the problems that can follow in the aftermath of the operation, including the following:

* loss of sex drive

* depression

* hair loss

* heart palpitations

* vaginal dryness and atrophy

* mood swings

* urinary tract infections

You may very well hear from your doctor, "Because you don't have a uterus, you can just take estrogen." But giving *unopposed* estrogen during this period can add more potential problems, such as weight gain, water retention, hypertension, blood clots, gallbladder disease, and breast and other cancers. Women who've had hysterectomies can end up spending even more time in the doctor's office dealing with a host of new ailments. The most frequent complaint of these women is weight gain. Over and over on the NWI hotline, we hear of women on Premarin after their hysterectomy who've gained twenty-five pounds and can't understand why and then can't exercise it off.

The idea that women with hysterectomies need only take estrogen to deal with a hormonal shortfall is not based on science. It is merely based on the idea that since you no longer have a uterus you are not at risk for endometrial cancer. But there are many reasons to supplement other hormones besides estrogen after a hysterectomy. The removal of the ovaries and uterus affects not only estrogen levels but also progesterone and testosterone levels, in addition to throwing a wrench in the balance of your whole endocrine system. In your body, estrogen is balanced by progesterone. They work in tandem. Replenishing progesterone can work against estrogen's effects on water retention and weight gain and can potentially protect against breast cancers, among its other major benefits.

There is also very good reason to replenish testosterone. More and more conventional doctors are using it as part of their HRT. Removal of the uterus and ovaries is a serious assault to your hormonal system. And "saving" the ovaries doesn't mean you will continue producing hormones as you did before the operation. After a hysterectomy the ovaries often stop functioning within two to three years. Testosterone replenishment has many benefits for a woman after a hysterectomy—including raising her energy and her libido, and maintaining and actually building bone.

Surgical Menopause Action Plan

* Get a baseline hormone test—for total estrogens (E1, E2, E3), progesterone, testosterone, and DHEA. For a woman in surgical menopause, it is particularly important to find a physician knowledgeable about natural hormones and who can work with her in establishing a program and monitoring its progress. (See the Natural Woman Institute referral service in the Resources section.)

* If you've just had the operation or are suffering severe symptoms, you should consider supplementing estradiol/progesterone and testosterone. You can then consider switching to a tri-est/progesterone formula, or later just progesterone alone, as your symptoms abate.

* See the advice in Chapter 2 on exercise and nutritional supplements.

* It is important for women with surgical menopause to keep a regular check on their bone density. Try to get an osteoporosis test once a year.

MENOPAUSE

The actual cessation of your period is a non-event. What is generally called menopause, with its related symptoms, can occur over a period as short as one year and as long as fifteen years, depending on the woman. Symptoms, however, are not inevitable. In fact, it's estimated that 25 percent of women pass through "the change" uneventfully and asymptomatically. These lucky women sail through this passage easily and wonder what others are complaining about.

A large number of women will have already experienced hormonal imbalance symptoms by the time their period actually stops, in the so-called perimenopausal period. The symptoms include hot flashes, night sweats, mood swings, foggy brain, fatigue, joint pain, anxiety, insomnia, and loss of sexual desire—and a woman can be completely relieved of them by age 55. Some women have hot flashes continuing intermittently for fifteen years. Some have them just a year or two.

Every woman will have her own unique experience. But one "symptom" seems to be true of almost all women: denial. Many working women, busy charging up the ladder, react to the first sign of menopause with terrible shock. Denial can then set in rapidly. But denial can become your enemy, as it can prevent you from dealing with symptoms, prolong discomfort unnecessarily, and, worst of all, prevent you from taking proper charge of your health. Put any denial behind you as soon as possible and stop all those bad habits that are accelerating your aging. The diet and exercise changes you make will be the most significant to your overall health and well-being. Many women with mild symptoms can control them with simple changes to exercise and diet.

Menopause is also very much a cultural phenomenon. In certain traditional cultures where old age is revered, women are less affected by the menopausal passage, both psychologically and symptomatically.

Why do Western women seem to have a greater incidence of menopausal symptoms, and why do women in Asian cultures have so few? Dr. Peter Ellison of Harvard University has studied women of menopausal age around the world. He believes that Western women have higher overall levels of estrogen, which reflects the fact that Western women eat both too much food and too little of what constitutes a healthy diet, and they don't exercise nearly enough. This lack of proper food intake and lack of exercise results in a higher risk for sex hormone–related cancers and more symptoms of hormonal imbalance, particularly when a woman reaches menopausal age. In American culture, it is undeniable that more and more women are experiencing hormone imbalance symptoms arising from increase in stress, dietary deficiencies, pollution, so-called xenoestrogens (harmful chemical substances in the environment that mimic or interfere with the body's hormones), and other factors that affect a woman's hormonal balance.

Regardless of the research, if you are a woman suffering menopausal symptoms, you want to know if hormone replacement is right for you. You have hot flashes and night sweats; your brain is foggy; you are tired all the time; sex is painful and you have no desire for it anyway. Your doctor may insist that you take Premarin/Provera to protect yourself against heart disease and osteoporosis. He or she says *you* have to make this decision. He or she says you have to protect your heart and your bones, but you are seriously worried about breast cancer, because you understand there is more risk for it with HRT.

First of all, you should consider menopause a wake-up call to take charge of your health. For a complete discussion of this issue, see *Natural Woman, Natural Menopause*. As to the safe and specific relief of menopausal symptoms, use the action plan that follows for the use of natural hormones. Once relieved of their symptoms, women get better than ever. Really! Above all, realize that you can come out of the passage healthier, stronger, full of vitality, and more beautiful than ever.

Menopause Action Plan

* If your symptoms are mild, consider a progesterone cream first. Some women do quite well using over-the-counter products.

* If the progesterone cream doesn't control your symptoms completely, you can use natural estrogen/progesterone for greater symptom relief. Testosterone can be helpful as well.

* See Chapter 5 (page 61) for information on adding testosterone to your hormone replenishment program.

* Follow the diet and exercise suggestions in Chapter 3. Read other books on health and fitness. Nothing will make you feel better than getting your body into shape, both inside and out.

AGING

A word about the cosmetic and anti-aging benefits of natural hormones. Needless to say, signs of aging are of genuine concern, and I believe that there is such a thing as healthy vanity. Using the natural hormones to restore normal levels can have revitalizing effects—on all the organs in your body, your immune system, your mood, your energy, and last but certainly not least, your libido.

I can attest to these numerous benefits personally. I look and feel younger than I did ten years ago. My face is fresh, firm, clear, and unlined (without a face lift!); my body is toned and strong. Today I take a combination of estrogen/progesterone/testosterone, with additional vitamin supplements and probiotics to protect my previously weakened intestinal tract. You deserve and can have no less.

POSTMENOPAUSE

When lecturing and on tour for *Natural Woman, Natural Menopause,* I would often meet women in their sixties and seventies who congratulated me on the book but then said that *they* didn't need to read it because they were past menopause. I would try to explain that it was a book for women of all ages—that all women need to know how their hormones work and put that knowledge to work for themselves for the enhancement of their well-being, and to protect themselves from wrong treatments that can quickly send them down the road to ill health and premature aging.

Some women think that after menopause, hormones have nothing to do with them. Not so. There are hormones in your body until you die. You continue to produce them, and they are still vital to how your body runs, so the balance is important. Excessively low levels may contribute to aging diseases such as Alzheimer's and Parkinson's. By using natural hormones judiciously, you can retard aging and change the quality of your life. After age 55, a woman is in the most danger of being given drugs she doesn't need—drugs that can trigger health problems, which can then put her into a cycle of never-ending ill health. It's important to educate yourself, if only to know what *not* to do.

One unfortunate scenario is that of a woman over 55 who has not menstruated for a few years and is feeling perfectly healthy, who goes to her doctor for an annual checkup. This doctor informs her that she has to take HRT drugs to protect herself against heart disease and osteoporosis. She begins taking the drugs, reacts to them badly, and finds herself newly miserable and feeling sick instead of well. So much for having an annual checkup.

Another unfortunate scenario is when a woman over seventy gets an osteoporosis test and her doctor puts her on Premarin/Provera, causing her to start bleeding! This is totally unnecessary! Using the natural hormones properly will not result in bleeding.

Recent studies have shown that high blood pressure can precipitate the onset of osteoporosis. This is but one of the many reasons a postmenopausal woman should learn all she can about controlling blood pressure with a proper diet. Expensive blood pressure medications can be avoided—in fact, many of the medications that women of a certain age believe to be their "fate" can be avoided.

Educating yourself about isoflavones (see page 73) can help you avoid dangerous osteoporosis drugs with many side effects. A new isoflavone product, Rimostil, was recently described at the North American Menopause Society's annual conference as a breakthrough in the search for a safe and effective therapy for women over 50 to help prevent osteoporosis and cardiovascular disease. That this conservative medical group is embracing the use of this isoflavone compound shows how far we have come toward breaking away from using estrogen drugs such as Premarin for their supposed long-term benefits. Rimostil has been shown to increase *cortical* bone—the bone involved in fractures—something that standard HRT drugs cannot do.

Judicious use of natural hormones postmenopause can allow you to remain healthy, vital, physically attractive, and sexually active for as long as you can. The great surge of attention to anti-aging therapies has sprung from the initial research about female hormones. There has been much media coverage of DHEA, melatonin, and HGH. Some of these therapies are still very experimental, but some will prove to have many benefits for people who want to remain healthy and vital well into old age.

Postmenopause Action Plan

* Get a baseline hormone test. You might want to consider replenishing hormones if your levels are low—in particular, testosterone for bone, libido, and overall energy, and progesterone for bone, skin, and potential cancer protection.

* Have an osteoporosis evaluation, both DEXA for bone density and Dpd for rate of bone loss. If necessary, begin taking progesterone for bone.

* Follow the guidelines for exercise, diet, and nutrition supplements in Chapter 3.

Part Two

YOUR QUESTIONS ANSWERED

Chapter Five

HORMONES AND YOUR BODY

*A*t every point in your life—from the onset of menstruation until old age—hormones will affect all aspects of your mental and physical well-being. Getting a firm grasp on the basics of how hormones work in your body will help you make intelligent choices about hormone replacement and give you a clear understanding of why you need to differentiate between natural and synthetic hormones.

What are hormones?

Hormones work as the "couriers" in your body. They deliver messages from your brain that tell your cells what to do—such as begin ovulation, go to sleep, or become aroused, to name but a few of their functions.

Think of the complex system of interdependent hormones in your body as a vastly sophisticated communications network that keeps your body working all day, every day. Hormones are continually circulating through your bloodstream, helping regulate all the crucial functions of your body.

Although there are many different kinds of hormones and even separate hormonal systems in the body, when talking about hormones in this book we are almost always talking about what are called *sex steroid hormones*. These hormones deal primarily with sexual functions and characteristics, but they also have thousands of other important functions.

The sex steroid hormones that most affect a woman's health, sexuality, and well-being are estrogen, progesterone, and testosterone. Other hormones that play an important but at this time less well-known role are pregnenolone, DHEA, and cortisol.

Your body makes its hormones from nutrients, with the aid of enzymes. The sex steroid hormones begin as a molecule of cholesterol. Cholesterol molecules transform into the hormone pregnenolone, which in turn transforms into progesterone, DHEA, testosterone, estrogen, and cortisol. The process by which one hormone transforms into another is described by scientists as a hormone *cascade*. A few other hormones are also involved in the overall sex steroid hormonal scheme, but for our purposes these six are all you need to know about.

When one hormone can transform into another, we say that it is a *precursor* to that hormone. Progesterone, for example, is a precursor for two other major sex hormones—estrogen and testosterone. This makes progesterone a particularly important hormone.

Sex hormones are constantly working with each other so that your hormonal makeup remains balanced. For example, if you have too much estrogen in your body, causing you to bloat and get headaches, your progesterone levels rise to counter these effects. During times when your natural balance is thrown off, such as during PMS, at menopause, and after having a baby, hormone replenishment can help restore balance.

How do hormones work?

Hormones essentially talk to each other to keep your body functioning. Think of them as "chemical messengers" moving through the bloodstream. The cells in every part of your body have *receptors* that bind only with specific hormones. Their purpose is to receive the messages the hormones are delivering. Receptors are very selective; with some exceptions, each will accept only its matching hormone. In other words, estrogen receptors will not bind with testosterone or DHEA molecules, only with estrogen molecules.

A specific hormone can instruct different parts of your body to do different things. If the target cell is a gland, for example, the instruction will be to secrete a specific substance at a specific time. In order for your hormone system to function smoothly, each receptor must exactly match up with its corresponding hormone. You could say they fit together like a lock and key.

In hormone replacement therapy, you add the hormones estrogen, progesterone, and testosterone to your bloodstream, where they attempt to attach to the correct receptors to do such things as lower anxiety, reduce hot flashes, and lift your mood. When things go wrong with standard HRT and you get negative side effects, it's usually because the synthetic HRT drugs (e.g. Premarin and Provera) are not exact matches for your receptors.

Another concern about synthetic hormones is that they cling to the receptor sites much longer than do your body's own hormones or natural hormones. After a hormone's message has been delivered, enzymes in the body begin to metabolize and then eliminate that hormone from your body. This process takes several hours with your body's hormones or the naturals. Some hormones foreign to your body, such as equilin (the horse estrogen in Premarin), can take eight to fourteen weeks to clear from your system because the body doesn't have the enzymes designed to handle this substance.

Because they cling so long to receptors, synthetic hormones can disturb the natural balancing functions of the various hormones in your body. If a synthetic hormone is attached to a receptor, other hormones can't attach there. As they linger in your body, the mismatched hormones may increase your risk of negative side effects and, in some cases, cancer.

What is a natural hormone?

The term *natural hormone* has come into use to differentiate it from synthetic and semisynthetic hormone products such as Premarin and Provera and other standard HRT drugs. Sometimes called *naturals*, these hormones are synthesized from wild yam or soy and match your own hormones exactly. They work in your body in the same manner as your own hormones and for this reason do not have the same side effects and long-term risk factors as do the standard HRT drugs. They are FDA-approved substances and have the same level of approval as Premarin and Provera, per FDA guidelines. Natural progesterone is available in low dose cream preparations over the counter. All other natural hormones are available by prescription from compounding pharmacists who make them to order. Unlike standard HRT drugs, natural hormones can be individualized (see Chapter 6, page 95, for a detailed description) to suit each woman's unique hormonal profile and needs.

What is a bio-identical plant-derived hormone?

The term *bio-identical plant-derived hormone* is a more specific term for a *natural hormone*. It is a hormone that is synthesized from either wild yam or soy and is biologically identical to the hormones produced in your body. It will function in your body in the exact same way as your body's hormones.

What's the difference between a synthesized hormone and a synthetic hormone?

The two terms are confusing, but there are very important distinctions between *synthetic* hormones and hormones that are *synthesized* from plants. Synthetic hormones mimic, but do not exactly match, human hormones. Synthetic hormones can be patented. Bio-identical plant-derived hormones, which are synthesized (in essence, distilled) from plants, cannot be patented, as they are exactly the same as substances that exist in nature. Patenting has a huge advantage in terms of the marketplace; drug companies can make large profits by selling patented products to which they have the exclusive rights. Hence, the general preference of drug companies up to now has been for synthetic substances.

With natural hormones, only the way in which they are delivered to the body (through a pill, patch, or cream) is patentable. These natural hormones exactly duplicate the body's own hormones, which makes them generally much safer and easier to metabolize than synthetic hormones.

What is a precursor hormone?

Looking at a diagram of what you could call the "sex steroid family tree" (see Figure 2), you will see that all sex hormones begin from a cholesterol molecule. From this starting point, the hormones form a *cascade* as one hormone transforms into another. Pregnenolone is a precursor to progesterone; progesterone is a precursor to testosterone and estrogens (E1, E2, E3). Looking at the way hormones are produced in your body, you can see how important it can be to pay attention to balancing your hormones, as some of these hormones can convert to each other as the body needs them. But adding too much of one hormone can leave your body without sufficient enzymes to metabolize other hormones completely.

What is estrogen?

Estrogen is not a single hormone, but a *family* of hormones produced by your body. There are at least two dozen estrogens, but the three most important are *estrone (E1), estradiol (E2),* and

FIGURE 2
Sex Steroid Hormone Cascade

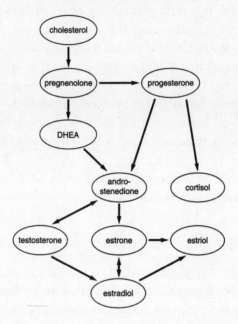

estriol (E3). Estrogen is produced primarily by your ovaries, but also by fat cells, muscle cells, and skin. Even after menopause, these sites continue to produce estrogen, albeit in different proportions.

Estrogen's main role in a woman's body is to spur the growth of female characteristics during puberty, to regulate the menstrual cycles, and to ensure the survival of a fetus. In cases where, for whatever reason (famine, anorexia nervosa, extreme athleticism), a woman has too little body fat to successfully carry a pregnancy to term, the estrogen levels in her body drop to prevent fertility. But in addition to the roles it plays regarding sex and procreation, estrogen also is responsible for at least *three hundred* other functions in your body. For instance, estrogen triggers the production of enzymes that support the connections between brain cells. It also affects your vision, hearing, taste, touch, and smell; your bones, heart, and skin; your mood; your sleep; your memory; your mental acuity and attention span; and your pain threshold. Estrogen doubtless plays many other roles that scientists have yet to discover.

The three main types of estrogen—estrone (E1), estradiol (E2), and estriol (E3)—have different properties and are produced in different amounts at different stages of your life.

Estradiol is considered the most active and powerful form of estrogen. It is produced primarily by your ovaries, beginning with your first menstrual cycle and tapering down at menopause. Estradiol and estrone (which converts to estradiol and vice versa) tend to promote cell division, which in turn can create a risk for endometrial, ovarian, and breast cancer. Of the three types of estrogen, estradiol is by far the most stimulating to cell growth in the breast— it is one thousand times more potent than estriol in this regard. Estradiol is the form of estrogen many doctors prefer for controlling hot flashes and other menopausal symptoms.

Estrone is usually converted from body fat and is the most common circulating hormone postmenopause. It is not considered as potent as estradiol but performs basically the same functions and behaves in the same way in your body. After menopause, your body is making more estrone than estradiol.

Estriol is made in large quantities by the placenta during pregnancy. In an average woman's body it is the largest circulating estrogen, as estradiol and estrone convert to estriol.

During pregnancy, the amount of estriol your body produces goes way up, while the quantity of estradiol and estrone dips much lower than normal. As noted previously, most of the circulating estrone and estradiol converts to estriol. Until recently, estriol was considered an unimportant *metabolite* (product) of the other estrogens, but recent research is demonstrating more important functions for it. Of the three main estrogens, only estriol is considered generally safe in terms of breast cancer risk. Studies have shown that estriol helps neutralize still-active estradiol and estrone by as much as 30 percent by competing with them for estrogen receptor sites, thus preventing them from stimulating these sites. As estradiol and estrone are more stimulating to breast tissue, this may be why some studies have shown that estriol may actually protect against breast cancer. It also has been shown to be a superior treatment for vaginal dryness and atrophy and urinary tract infections.

What's the difference between natural plant-derived estrogen and synthetic estrogen?

Natural plant-derived estrogen is synthesized from wild yam or soy. Its molecular structure exactly duplicates the structure of the body's own estradiol, estrone, or estriol. Because it is natural—that is, bio-identical—it can deliver the same benefits to your body as your own estrogen, without the uncomfortable side effects associated with synthetic estrogen.

Synthetic estrogens are created from various sources, such as horse urine or plants. The most widely used synthetic estrogen is Premarin, which is composed of 52 percent horse estrogens (a match only for horses) and 48 percent estrone (which matches human estrone). In synthetics that use a plant base, the molecular structure has been slightly altered. This altered structure of synthetic estrogen can result in unpleasant side effects and health risks for women who use them.

My doctor says Premarin is natural because it's made from horse urine, which comes from nature. Is he right?

It's true that synthetic products such as Premarin are made from so-called natural ingredients, such as horse urine. Even Provera, a synthetic drug with many unpleasant side effects, is a molecularly altered version of natural progesterone.

Nevertheless, synthetic hormones are considered unnatural. This is because the synthetic's molecular structure does not match the natural structure of the body's hormones. The "natural" designation refers to how it acts in the body, not to its source.

Synthetic hormones do not behave in the body the way your own hormones would. In the case of Provera, a pharmaceutical company altered a few molecules of natural progesterone, making the drug unique and therefore patentable. But those few molecules created a substantial mismatch between Provera and the body's natural progesterone. In the case of Premarin, equilin—one of the horse estrogens it contains—does not match human estrogen. Neither drug is a natural match to your body's own hormones. The manufacturers of these products present them as "estrogen" and "progesterone"; unfortunately, this has contributed mightily to the confusion and controversy surrounding HRT drugs.

What are the possible side effects of Premarin?

Long-term risks include cancer of the uterus, cancer of the breast, gallbladder disease, and abnormal blood clotting. Side effects include nausea and vomiting, breast tenderness or enlargement, enlargement of benign tumors of the uterus, retention of excess fluid (which may worsen some conditions such as asthma, epilepsy, migraine, heart disease, or kidney disease), and a spotty darkening of the skin.

I suggest you check for yourself all the contraindications for the use of Premarin in the *Physicians' Desk Reference* (available at your library or on the Internet at *www.pdrnet.com*), as they would be impossible to reprint in this small space.

I've heard the phrase estrogen dominance. *What does it mean?*

This phrase was coined by Dr. John Lee, a leading expert in natural hormones and author of *What Your Doctor May* Not *Tell You About Menopause,* and is a very useful way of describing what can happen when estrogen and progesterone get out of balance in your body. Estrogen dominance doesn't mean there is too much estrogen in your system, but rather that there is too much estrogen *in relation to progesterone.* Women in menopause continue to make estrogen in muscle and fat cells. Typically, such a woman produces 40 to 60 percent of the estrogen she produced before menopause, but produces only $\frac{1}{120}$ of the progesterone. So even though she has less estrogen than she did before menopause, she is still estrogen dominant: There is not enough progesterone in her system to counter the effects of the estrogen that remains. During perimenopause, when a woman's estrogen levels tend to spike up and down, she becomes estrogen dominant—too much estrogen at certain times in relation to her progesterone. Adding more estrogen can make this condition worse.

What is tri-estrogen?

Tri-estrogen (tri-est) is a combination formula of the three types of estrogen—estrone (E1), estradiol (E2), and estriol (E3)—in a 1:1:8 ratio. The idea behind this formula is to balance the estradiol and estrone, with their more powerful stimulating effects, with the weaker but more potentially protective estriol. Estradiol is twelve times more potent than estrone and eighty times more potent than estriol in terms of the estrogenic impact on your body. Estradiol is a great help in alleviating hot flashes, night sweats, and other menopause symptoms, but it also carries a higher risk for breast cancer. As noted on page 73, estriol has been shown in some studies to protect against breast cancer. The tri-est formula is an attempt to get the benefits of all three estrogens while minimizing possible cancer risks. Dr. Jonathan Wright, an early pioneer in the use of natural hormones, created this formula based on the fact that the 1:1:8 ratio represents the average normal amounts of circulating estrogen in a 35-year-old woman.

Even though tri-est is generally considered safer than estradiol alone, standard protocol is still to take it with progesterone, for balance and for even more cancer protection. Some doctors use only estradiol/progesterone for hormone replacement, believing that when estradiol is used with progesterone, cell proliferation in both the uterus and the breast is sufficiently curbed. The estradiol/progesterone formula is frequently recommended for women who've just had a hysterectomy, as they often need more estradiol to combat symptoms, at least in the short term.

What is bi-estrogen?

Whereas tri-est contains all three primary types of estrogen—estradiol, estriol, and estrone—bi-est contains only two: estradiol and estriol. The bi-est formula is 80 percent estriol, 20 percent estradiol. Like tri-est, bi-est is available by prescription through a compounding pharmacy. It was recently developed as an alternative to tri-est (see page 70) by certain doctors who felt that given the interactivity of estradiol and estrone, and the fact that most estrone is produced as a woman gets older, it was unnecessary to provide estrone as part of the formula. You would take bi-est just as you would tri-est, in that you would always balance it with progesterone.

What is a phytoestrogen?

A phytoestrogen is a plant compound that exerts an estrogen-like effect in your body. Phytoestrogens work either by mimicking estrogenic activities—they are known to bind with estrogen receptors—or by helping your body regulate its own estrogen. Phytoestrogens are not the same as natural hormones. Natural hormones as described in this book are synthesized from wild yam or soy and exactly match your own hormones.

Even though phytoestrogens are not technically hormones, they can be powerful agents for alleviating discomfort. For centuries, women have used herbal remedies containing phytoestrogens not only for menopause but for PMS, pregnancy and delivery, menstrual cramps, dysmenorrhea (lack of periods), and other "female ailments."

Black cohosh is probably the most popular and widely tested herbal remedy containing phytoestrogens. Others that have gained some recognition in the United States are dong quai, wild yam, and chaste tree berry. You can purchase most of these at health food stores or through mail order companies; large cities almost certainly have shops that specialize in herbal remedies. Remifemin (see Chapter 10, page 131) is made from black cohosh and is available at most stores or by mail order. (See the Resources section.)

Phytoestrogens are part of a larger classification called *phytohormones* (also known as *phytochemicals, phytonutrients,* and *nutraceuticals*). *Phytohormone* is a broad term used to describe any plant compound that has a hormonelike effect on your system. Researchers have discovered more than three hundred plants that contain phytoestrogens or phytoprogesterones. Legumes, grains, nuts, and seeds are especially good sources. These foods can sometimes help alleviate symptoms of PMS or menopause. They are also important to both men and women for their general health benefits. We need these plant foods for both their nutritional and hormone-balancing properties. A plant-based diet is considered fundamental to cancer protection. The phytohormone *diosgenin,* from which natural hormones are derived, is found in a tropical wild yam. Natural hormones are also derived from *genistein,* found in soy.

What are isoflavones? Are they hormones?

Isoflavones are phytoestrogens found in a variety of legumes, particularly soybeans. They produce a weak estrogenic effect in the body, which some women find helpful in alleviating menopausal symptoms.

Since 1993, more than a thousand studies have been published concerning isoflavones. The studies show that isoflavones benefit women in three main areas: They minimize cell damage from free radicals, inhibit tumor cell growth, and protect against breast cancer. This last finding is especially exciting for women who need relief from menopause symptoms but are at risk for breast cancer. Isoflavones protect the breasts by attaching to the receptor sites upon which estrogen molecules land—in other words, they occupy the estrogen's space. Estrogen (particularly estradiol) has been linked to increased risk of breast cancer. Isoflavones limit the number of receptor sites available to estrogens, while still providing positive estrogen-like effects such as relief from hot flashes.

You can get isoflavones either from eating foods that are rich in them, such as soy, chickpeas, lentils, and beans, or by taking an isoflavone dietary supplement such as Promensil. You'd have to eat a lot of legumes (for instance, 10 cups of chickpeas) to equal the 40 milligrams of isoflavones contained in a Promensil tablet. But bear in mind that some researchers claim one serving of soy milk or tofu contains "therapeutic" levels of isoflavones. No one has yet determined an ideal dosage of isoflavones, and new studies are being done every year.

I've been told that estriol protects against breast cancer. Is this true?

In 1966, the *Journal of the American Medical Association* (*JAMA*) published a report by H. M. Lemon, M.D., who had discovered a correlation between higher levels of estriol and remission of breast cancer. Dr. Lemon also studied women without breast cancer and found that they had naturally higher estriol levels, compared with estrone and estradiol levels, than women with breast cancer.

Another article, published in *JAMA* in 1978 and appropriately titled "Estriol, The Forgotten Estrogen," provided more evidence for estriol's protective properties. In the article, A. H. Follingstad, M.D., reported on his use of estriol as a treatment for breast cancer. Follingstad had administered small doses of estriol to postmenopausal women with breast cancer. Thirty-seven percent of the women experienced either a remission of the cancer or arrest of their cancerous lesions.

All estrogens promote cell division in breast tissue, which in turn can increase the risk of breast cancer. However, estradiol and estrone stimulate the tissue far more than estriol does. Many researchers believe that estriol may protect against breast cancer by occupying receptor sites that otherwise would be taken by estrone.

What is progesterone?

Progesterone is a hormone of the reproductive system. When an egg is released from your ovary, it leaves behind ruptured follicles called the *corpus luteum* ("yellow body"), from which progesterone is produced. In pregnant women, the placenta also produces progesterone. In fact, the name *progesterone* comes from the word *progestation*.

Two of the primary functions of progesterone in pregnancy are to prepare the lining of the uterus for implantation of a fertilized egg and then to ensure the survival of a fetus. But progesterone has also been shown in recent research to have important functions for the nervous system (maintaining nerve cells, motor function, and sense of touch), the brain, and the bones. It has been shown to actually build new bone, as opposed to estrogen, which has only been shown to halt bone loss. Progesterone is also a precursor hormone, which means that it transforms to create other hormones, including estrogen and testosterone. This precursor function makes progesterone a very important player in terms of overall hormone balance. When your body has an adequate supply of progesterone, it has the flexibility to create the various hormones it needs. When progesterone levels drop, the body loses some of its ability to quickly create other hormones.

Progesterone also *opposes* the estrogen in your system, meaning that it balances some of the more intense and undesirable effects of estrogen. For instance, estradiol is known to cause cells in the breast to grow, creating a high risk for breast cancer. Progesterone can cancel out this estrogenic effect. Unopposed estrogen, whether produced by your own body or introduced in the form of HRT, can increase the risk for endometrial cancer, breast cancer, and a host of other afflictions. Unopposed estrogen can:

* cause water retention

* cause high blood pressure

* reduce oxygen in the cells

* oppose thyroid function

* promote histamine release, causing allergy-type symptoms

* promote blood clotting, which can lead to a higher risk of stroke and embolism

* promote gallbladder disease

* decrease sex drive

By opposing these effects of estrogen, progesterone plays a vital role in maintaining your health and well-being. In addition, progesterone:

* can improve sleep

* has a natural calming effect during the day

* can eliminate water retention and weight gain by balancing out the properties of estrogen

* improves the body's ability to use and eliminate fats

* appears to have a positive effect against hypertension

* stimulates new bone formation (unlike estradiol, which so far has been shown only to retard bone loss)

* may protect against breast cancer

* normalizes your sex drive

* can regrow scalp hair in women

When women enter menopause, their progesterone is reduced more than their estrogen, proportionally speaking. That's why it's so important for any HRT regimen to include progesterone along with estrogen, and why in many cases replacing progesterone alone is enough to alleviate menopausal symptoms.

What is the difference between natural progesterone and synthetic progestins?

Progesterone is a hormone made by your body. A *progestin* is a synthetic form of progesterone; its molecular structure does not match the structure of your body's progesterone. Provera is one of the many progestins on the market today. (Provera is the progestin used in Prempro and Premphase.) Progesterone that is synthesized from either wild yam or soy (frequently called "natural" progesterone to set it apart from progestin) matches human progesterone exactly—it is bio-identical. Progestin is much more potent than progesterone. It was originally developed for use in birth control pills, where a stronger form of progesterone was needed to interrupt the menstrual cycle.

At one time, doctors believed there was no discernible difference between your body's natural progesterone and the synthetic progestins. Even today, many physicians and members of the media wrongly assume that the two hormone substances are identical. But by opting to use synthetic progestin instead of natural progesterone in hormone replacement therapy, drug manufacturers ended up shortchanging the women they hoped to help.

Current research shows that progestin and progesterone behave quite differently in a woman's body. Progesterone is a precursor hormone, meaning that the body uses it to create other essential hormones such as estrogen and testosterone. Progestins, on the other hand, cannot help the body produce or balance hormones. In fact, progestins can actually inhibit the body's progesterone precursor functions.

Where most women notice the difference between progesterone and progestin are in side effects. Natural progesterone has many positive side effects, as listed in the previous question. Progestin has none of these beneficial properties. Not only does it interfere with progesterone's precursor functions, but progestin can also cause a host of unpleasant side effects (see below). And although progestin does protect against endometrial cancer, it does not have progesterone's potential protective benefit to the breast.

What are the possible side effects of progestins such as Provera?

The 1999 *Physicians' Desk Reference*, which lists the side effects and contraindications of all pharmaceuticals sold in the

United States, includes the following among possible side effects of progestin:

* breast tenderness

* edema

* rashes

* acne

* hirsutism (increased hair growth)

* weight changes (increase or decrease)

* depression

* nausea

* insomnia

* somnolence

* severe acute allergic reaction

* breakthrough bleeding, spotting, amenorrhea, or changes in menses

* thrombophlebitis and pulmonary embolism

* cervical erosions and changes in cervical secretions

* cholestatic jaundice

When taken with estrogens (for example, Premarin), the following may occur:

* headaches

* dizziness

* rise in blood pressure

* fatigue

* nervousness

* changes in sex drive

* loss of scalp hair or hirsutism

* PMS-like symptoms

* urinary tract infections

* itchiness

Does natural progesterone protect against endometrial cancer?

When used in hormone replacement therapy, *both* natural progesterone and synthetic progestin (for example, Provera) protect against endometrial cancer.

Does natural progesterone carry the same cancer risks as Provera?

A 1995 Harvard study claimed a link between the use of Premarin/Provera and increased risk of breast cancer. The researchers found that the use of estrogen replacement pills (the study used Premarin) increased a woman's risk of breast cancer by 30 percent, and that if she also used Provera the risk went up to 40 percent.

Unfortunately, because many physicians and members of the media mistakenly believe that natural progesterone and Provera are the same, there have been false claims that "progesterone" causes an increased risk of breast cancer. But the Harvard study dealt exclusively with Premarin and Provera, not with natural estrogen and progesterone. A leading menopause specialist at Vanderbilt University, Dr. Joel Hargrove, has suggested that until natural hormones are used in testing, the results of hormone studies remain inconclusive and misleading.

To date there is no evidence that the use of natural progesterone increases a woman's risk of breast cancer. In fact, recent studies indicate that progesterone may *protect against* breast cancer. The most important of these studies was published in the April 1995 *Journal of Fertility and Sterility*. It showed that natural, plant-derived progesterone inhibits estrogen's stimulation of normal breast tissue cells. This cell stimulation can lead to breast cancer.

The bottom line: Current research shows that both Provera and natural progesterone protect against endometrial cancer. Provera, when used with Premarin, has been shown to increase a woman's risk of breast cancer. Natural progesterone has not been shown to increase the risk of breast cancer, and may well protect against it.

Do natural hormones lower "bad" cholesterol (LDL) and raise "good" cholesterol (HDL)?

Natural estrogen has the same beneficial effects on cholesterol levels that have been touted for Premarin in an important study called the PEPI (Postmenopausal Estrogen/Progestin Intervention) trial, published in 1995, which showed that when Provera, a synthetic, was added to estrogen, the cholesterol-lowering effects were actually reduced by 30 percent! But when natural progesterone was added, it didn't diminish in any statistically significant way the positive effects on lowering bad cholesterol and raising good cholesterol. The natural progesterone showed itself to be a far better balancing and protective agent than estrogen. However, bear in mind that reducing cholesterol levels does not necessarily translate in a one-to-one fashion as protection against heart disease. Many cholesterol-lowering drugs have not been found to reduce the risk of heart disease, and some have actually increased the risk.

What is testosterone?

Testosterone is a sex steroid hormone produced by both men and women—although in much smaller amounts in women. Until recently, its importance to a woman's body has been underestimated and ignored. Among its functions in your body are accelerating tissue growth and stimulating blood flow. Women produce testosterone mainly in their ovaries; smaller amounts are made in the adrenals. Its levels decline as they age. When prescribed in menopause, it can improve libido, build new bone, and improve energy, alertness, and well-being.

For women who have had a hysterectomy and therefore an abrupt interruption in hormone production, testosterone can be particularly beneficial. When it is prescribed in low, regulated doses, women can usually gain the benefits and avoid the negative side effects of too much testosterone, such as acne and hair growth on the face.

What is DHEA?

DHEA (dehydroepiandrosterone) is a steroid hormone manufactured primarily in the adrenal glands. It is a precursor (see Chapter 5, page 62) to testosterone and estrogen, and is important to the building and repair of protein in the body. Because its levels decline with age, it is seen as an important marker for aging. Until recently, its function and importance in the body were not well understood, but in many people DHEA has been known to increase well-being and boost energy, and it may help protect against osteoporosis. If you're interested in using it, get a hormone test, either blood or saliva, to keep track of your levels. I suggest obtaining prescription DHEA and staying away from over-the-counter products, particularly those that advertise themselves as DHEA precursors, as there is no evidence that they work. If you're already taking testosterone, you may want to forgo DHEA, as it converts to testosterone and some women have experienced testosterone-like side effects, such as acne and growth of facial hair, with its use.

What is pregnenolone?

Pregnenolone is a precursor (see Chapter 5, page 62) to all the other sex steroid hormones and is made in all the cells of the body except red blood cells. Its potential benefits when used in hormone replacement therapy are less well-known than the other steroid hormones. Theoretically, it would seem possible to take pregnenolone itself, thereby providing the body with what it needs to make all the other steroid hormones. But monitoring of hormone levels has shown this to be false. There is also some preliminary evidence that pregnenolone supplementation can benefit rheumatoid arthritis symptoms and increase brain cell activity.

What is cortisol? Is it a hormone?

Cortisol is a steroid hormone—meaning it is produced from cholesterol—and although it is technically not a *sex* steroid hormone, I am including it because it interacts with other sex steroid hormones, particularly DHEA. Although cortisol has many functions in the body, it is the primary hormone when it comes to regulating stress. When you're under stress, whether it's emotional stress or physical stress—such as infection, pain, or intense exercise—your adrenal glands secrete extra cortisol. High levels of stress over long periods of time lead to high levels of cortisol in the blood, which make a demand on both progesterone and DHEA to maintain balance. In this way, stress can have a negative effect on your hormonal balance.

What is a xenoestrogen?

A *xenoestrogen* (also called a *xenobiotic* or *xenohormone*) is a chemical substance in the environment that can mimic and/or interfere with your body's own hormones. They are principally found in the petrochemicals, including pesticides and solvents, that are now so abundant in our lives. They can invisibly affect you in the form of hormonal imbalances, birth defects, decreased libido, and cancers, principally breast and prostate cancer. The prevalence of xenoestrogen and other threats to your hormonal health is why I'm recommending that you protect yourself with the right diet, concentrating on plant-based foods and additional nutritional supplements (see Chapter 3, page 29).

How does diet affect my hormones?

There is a direct, crucial link between the food you eat and your hormonal makeup. Put simply, the more vegetables and fewer animal fats you ingest, the more likely you are to enjoy hormonal balance and overall good health.

Vegetables rich in phytohormones raise or lower your body's hormone levels as needed. Eating too many animal fats, on the other hand, can create a hormonal imbalance and raise your estrogen levels. This increases your risk of breast cancer and other cancers. What's more, there is some evidence that excess fat in the diet adversely affects the way hormones interact with one another.

In addition to being good for your hormones, a plant-rich diet is excellent preventive medicine for many of today's most common diseases. An overwhelming number of studies—at least 150 around the world—have determined that people who eat the most fruits and vegetables are half as likely to have cancer as people who eat the least. A low–animal-fat diet also is standard protocol for anyone with heart disease, since fat raises cholesterol.

For women in perimenopause or menopause, a plant-based diet can have a tremendous impact on well-being and severity of symptoms. Perhaps nothing can make this point more bluntly than the fact that in Japan, where the traditional diet consists primarily of soy foods and vegetables, there is no word for *hot flashes*. A plant-based diet does such a good job of regulating a woman's hormones that menopausal symptoms are practically unknown there. Soy, in particular, is believed to be a prime reason for the high quality of hormonal health in Japanese women. The Japanese typically eat 50 to 80 grams of soy per day, whereas Americans eat about 5 grams—usually in the form of salad dressing or other foods loaded with fats and preservatives. Studies have shown that when Asian women move to the West and begin to eat a Western diet, they too start having menopausal symptoms.

It's not necessary for you to forgo meat entirely to benefit from a plant-rich diet. However, the more vegetables you eat, the better your chance of maintaining a well-balanced system without having to take additional hormones of any kind. Legumes, grains, nuts, and seeds are all good sources of phytohormones. Soy, especially in fermented forms such as miso and tempeh, is probably the best source of all. Fifty to 80 grams, by the way, is only about 2 to 3 ounces.

How does digestion affect hormone levels?

A well-functioning digestive system efficiently absorbs nutrients from the food you eat. This is crucial to your hormonal balance, because your body needs nutrients to convert one hormone to another. Poor digestion, then, can hamper your body's ability to convert hormones. If you are taking natural hormones orally, poor digestion may also hinder their absorption.

In addition, bad digestion can lead to an imbalance of your *intestinal flora*—microbes that are responsible for making antibodies and utilizing vitamins, among other tasks. When the intestinal flora are imbalanced, they sometimes convert estrogen that should be eliminated into a form that can be reabsorbed, which in turn can put you at risk for estrogen-sensitive cancers.

A number of telltale signs indicate that your digestive tract is not functioning as smoothly as it could be:

* heartburn

* ulcers

* indigestion

* gas

* constipation

* diarrhea

* bloating

* inability to each much at one sitting

* feeling "full" long after a meal has ended

Unfortunately, the antacids we often take to combat these ailments are not beneficial to our hormones. Antacids can interfere with our ability to use the phytoestrogens in the food we eat. (Phytoestrogens are plant compounds that exert an estrogenlike effect in the body.) The new generation of over-the-counter stomach remedies—"H2 blockers" such as Tagamet, Zantac, and Pepcid—are harmful for a different reason: They interfere with the absorption of nutrients, especially calcium.

Antacids and H2 blockers can provide immediate relief from pain, but the next day—or meal—usually brings another round of discomfort. Taking antacids after every meal, or as one company suggests, taking an H2 blocker before your meal, cannot improve your digestive system. The only way to do that is to change your diet. A great many people can be completely cured of their stomach problems by changing what they eat and perhaps taking plant digestive enzyme supplements.

Certain foods are known to be hard on your digestive tract. Any effective treatment plan will require you to eliminate these from your diet, at least until all is running smoothly again:

* coffee

* citrus fruits

* tomatoes and tomato-based foods

* spicy foods

* alcohol

* fried foods

* extremely fatty foods

* chocolate

* overly sweet foods

For heartburn and ulcer conditions, coffee (including decaf) is a prime culprit. Do away with coffee for a few weeks and see if it makes a difference.

Three other elements are also known to exacerbate digestive disorders. Certain prescription drugs—principally painkillers—irritate the stomach; if you are taking any, ask your doctor to check on this. Perhaps the prescription can be changed. Smoking, too, can cause stomach upset. The nicotine in cigarette smoke can increase heartburn and cause you to burp up stomach acid, so stop smoking or cut back as much as possible. Finally, stress can be a factor. Stress affects everyone differently, and some people "take it in the gut"—their stomach clenches, the juices start roiling, and pain soon follows. If you get no relief from dietary changes and supplements, and you aren't smoking or taking prescription drugs, stress may be at the root of your stomach problems.

There are natural solutions to digestion problems. Plant digestive enzyme supplements aid your stomach's digestive enzymes, which are responsible for breaking food down into nutrients. The plant enzymes come in capsules and are available over the counter at health food stores and some pharmacies. The following are some popular brands:

Prevail's Vitase Digestion Formula

Rainbow Light's Advance Enzyme System

Futurebiotics Vegetarian Enzyme Complex

Tyler Encapsulations Similase

Although these supplements are safe to use over the long term, you won't necessarily have to. Start by taking two to four capsules before each meal. Ideally, you'll be ridding your diet of the foods listed earlier, so your meals will be gentler on the stomach. After two months, if you're feeling a lot better, you can stop taking the enzymes and see if you maintain improved digestion.

If you suffer from an ulcer or pre-ulcerous condition such as chronic gastritis (symptoms include heartburn and acid indigestion), don't start taking the digestive enzymes right away. Instead, begin with a product called Acid-Ease, made by Prevail. After two months, gradually switch from the Acid-Ease to the enzymes. Naturally, if you have severe and chronic digestive problems, you should consult a doctor.

What are the benefits of natural hormones?

The benefits of natural hormones fall into two main categories: They alleviate unpleasant symptoms of PMS, perimenopause, and menopause; and they help protect against certain diseases.

Natural hormones can help alleviate the following:

* depression, anxiety, and other mood swings

* hot flashes

* night sweats

* cramping

* headaches

* bloating

* sore breasts

* insomnia

* low sex drive

* thinning skin

* vaginal wall thinning and dryness; painful intercourse

* hair loss

* postpartum depression

Long-term benefits include possible protection against the following:

* heart disease

* osteoporosis—progesterone can build bone

* breast cancer

* Alzheimer's disease

In addition, there are long-term cosmetic benefits to hair, nails, and skin.

Can hormone replenishment prevent Alzheimer's disease?

The news on this front is encouraging. A number of studies have indicated that taking estrogen does reduce the risk of Alzheimer's. In the June 1997 issue of *Neurology,* researchers from the National Institute on Aging in Bethesda and Johns Hopkins Bayview Medical Center in Baltimore reported that women who take estrogen after menopause reduce their risk of Alzheimer's by 50 percent. The study involved 472 women who had been observed for more than sixteen years.

Earlier research also pointed to estrogen's beneficial effect on the brain. One study indicated that estrogen can inhibit age-related deterioration of brain cells by acting as an anti-inflammatory and antioxidant agent. Estrogen also has been shown to spur the growth of neurons that release acetylcholine, which transmits nerve messages in the brain.

The Women's Health Initiative, a government research project, is currently conducting long-term studies that will establish the extent to which estrogen can protect the brain from Alzheimer's. The results of that study will not be available until sometime in the next ten years, but meanwhile there seems to be strong evidence that estrogen can lower the risk of Alzheimer's. If you have a family history of the disease, it would be worth your while to research this topic. There are many ways to do this on the Internet. HealthWorld Online (*www.healthy.net*) is an excellent resource and provides free access to the Medline database, which lists all the latest research breakthroughs relating to Alzheimer's disease.

Will natural hormones improve my skin?

Natural hormones can be helpful in improving your skin in several ways.

Some women, when they reach their late thirties to early forties, have a resurgence of that old teenage nemesis, acne. The reasons for this are unclear (although it is likely that it is hormone related), but many women have found that a topical progesterone cream is helpful in clearing up the condition. There is also evidence to suggest that topical progesterone cream can alleviate *seborrhea,* a condition that causes flaking, itching skin.

Women in menopause commonly complain that their skin has lost its tone and youthful glow. Three hormones—estrogen, progesterone, and testosterone—have been linked to this problem. (There is also some evidence that points to DHEA having a positive effect on wrinkles.) Estrogen and progesterone both contribute to healthy skin, and since they decrease at menopause, it's no surprise that some women notice a difference in skin tone after "the change." Testosterone levels drop by almost half during menopause. Some research indicates that this decrease in testosterone can lead to a number of symptoms, including thin, dry skin. However, be wary of replacing too much testosterone, as it can cause facial hair growth and acne.

There are essentially two ways your skin can benefit from natural hormones: from the inside and from the outside. If you are in menopause and experiencing thinning and/or dry skin, replenishing hormones—both estrogen and progesterone—will benefit you. In addition, both these hormones can be helpful to your skin when used topically. Progesterone in particular is used in skin creams to great effect. And the use of a skin cream with *alphahydroxy acids*—also known as *fruit acids*—can slough off dead cells and clarify your skin. Over-the-counter products with alphahydroxy acids usually contain no more than 2 to 3 percent. Generally, you need an 8 to 10 percent concentration to get a good effect. A facialist or dermatologist can make up a cream for you. When you feel a slight tingly sensation, it is doing its job. Then, if you add exercise, a proper diet, and plenty of water, your skin will be glowing, toned, and youthful-looking again.

My hair is thinning. Will natural hormones help?

One of the side effects of decreased levels of progesterone can be thinning hair. This is because progesterone is a precursor to a number of adrenal cortical hormones. Progesterone is produced primarily in the ovaries. When the ovaries are no longer functioning, progesterone levels drop, and the body must find an alternate precursor for the adrenal cortical hormones. *Androstenedione* is that alternate precursor. The body produces more of it in response to the lack of progesterone.

The problem is, androstenedione can promote masculine properties in women—for example, male-pattern hair loss. Replacing natural progesterone should solve the problem in many cases, but it can take up to six months to see results. Hair growth, even in young women, is a slow process.

Women who have had hysterectomies also frequently experience hair loss, which is a reason that replacement therapy should include progesterone as well as estrogen.

When I look in the mirror, I see the beginnings of middle-age spread. Do hormones have anything to do with this? Can taking natural hormones help?

The research in this area is fairly new; for the first time, women are getting reasonable explanations for the weight gain that begins to creep in around age 40. Middle-age spread, it turns out, is at least partly related to your ovaries' drop in estrogen production.

Women have about thirty billion fat cells, which perform a variety of functions in the body. One of these is to produce estrogen. Prior to perimenopause, your ovaries produce most of the estrogen your body needs. When the ovaries begin to slow their estrogen production, your fat cells increase their production to take up the slack. It's your body's attempt to maintain hormonal balance. To increase estrogen production, the number of fat cells multiplies, the cells get bigger (by at least 20 percent), and they actually increase their ability to store fat. According to Debra Waterhouse, author of *Outsmarting the Mid-Life Fat Cell*, "The fat cells in your waist grow the largest because they are better equipped to produce estrogen than the fat cells in your buttocks, hips, and thighs." This accounts for the spreading waistline that is a particular source of anguish to so many women.

Some studies on HRT and weight gain indicate that women on HRT gain more fat in the lower body than women who don't take hormones; a European study found that the size of fat cells in the thigh increased by 50 percent in women on HRT. Another study found that HRT didn't necessarily affect the *amount* of weight women gained in menopause, but that it did affect *where* the weight was gained: Women on HRT were more likely to gain in their lower body than women who were not taking hormones.

Whether you take natural hormones, traditional HRT, or no hormone therapy at all, odds are that you'll gain some weight before and during menopause. In addition to your fat cells working overtime, your metabolism also slows at midlife. As Waterhouse explains, "Muscle is your metabolism, and when you lose muscle, you lose your ability to burn calories. . . . From age 35 on, the average woman loses about a pound and a half of muscle a year while she's gaining one-and-a-half pounds of fat. When you lose a half pound of muscle, you burn forty fewer calories a day. The more muscle you lose, the fewer calories your body needs, and the extra calories are rerouted to your fat cells to store."

This double whammy—slower metabolism and increased number and size of fat cells—causes middle-age spread. A weight gain of up to ten pounds is generally considered OK; any more than that, and your health may be compromised. Gaining thirty pounds or more has been associated with increased risk of breast cancer and heart disease.

During perimenopause and menopause, it's especially crucial that you eat a healthy diet. You should also accept the fact that it may be impossible to lose that final five or ten pounds until you're past menopause. Your best bet for controlling your weight is to exercise—support your muscles and burn calories (and lose fat) by maintaining a faster metabolism.

The good news is that around age 55, when you're through "the change," your fat cells make another transition: They slow their estrogen production and stop storing so much fat. The cells actually shrink in size, and you become able to lose weight more easily again.

Can taking hormones give me more energy?

Fatigue and insomnia are symptoms of menopause, and women in perimenopause are apt to experience fatigue and morning sluggishness. There seems to be a connection between fatigue and hormonal fluctuations, but researchers have yet to discover the exact nature of that connection.

In his book *What Your Doctor May Not Tell You About Menopause,* Dr. John Lee reports successfully treating patients with natural progesterone to mitigate fatigue and poor sleep patterns. He also sites a study by Eric Braverman, Ph.D. (reported in *Total Health,* August 1993), which indicates that increased sleepiness is the one discernible side effect of natural progesterone. For this reason, Dr. Lee suggests that his patients apply progesterone cream (or take their oral dose) just prior to bedtime.

If your fatigue is due to insomnia or poor sleep patterns, natural progesterone may help by giving you a better night's sleep. If hot flashes have been keeping you up, alleviating them may be the solution. Natural hormones, including some tri-est or estradiol if necessary, will probably do the trick.

But what if the opposite is true—you're sleeping *too* well and never seem able to "get with it"? In that case, I recommend that you get your hormone levels tested and begin taking natural progesterone (and estrogen) if the levels warrant it. Even though we don't fully understand why hormones affect our energy level, the fact that fatigue is a symptom of both menopause and perimenopause indicates that hormones are related to the problem. Balancing your hormones may therefore help raise your energy level.

In addition, you should consider adding testosterone to your hormone replenishment regime. Testosterone is known to increase energy levels and a sense of well-being—not to mention your libido. More and more conventional doctors are prescribing testosterone along with estrogen in their HRT regimes.

Chapter Six

USING NATURAL HORMONES

Natural hormones are readily available. There are compounding pharmacies in nearly every major city, and the large mail-order compounders who specialize in natural hormones fill prescriptions by mail (see the Resources section for a complete listing). But to reap the most benefits from the naturals, you need to know all your options. Once you understand the terminology and are aware of the various types of hormones and how they are administered, you can have a confident, informed discussion with your doctor. Together, the two of you can develop a treatment that meets all your needs.

How can I get natural hormones?

Natural hormones are available in two ways: by prescription sold at compounding pharmacies or in preformulated package products sold over the counter (primarily at health food stores). If you and your doctor have decided to use over-the-counter products, there are progesterone creams and tri-est/progesterone creams available, but the strength is limited to 2 percent. Prescription natural hormones can be formulated to order in strengths prescribed by your doctor. They are available in a wide variety of forms: creams, pills, drops, sublinguals (dissolved under the tongue), patches, and suppositories.

How do I take natural hormones—or what's a "delivery system"?

A delivery system is the means by which a substance is delivered to your body. In the United States, the delivery systems we are most accustomed to are oral (pills) and injection. Transdermals ("through the skin") are becoming more widely used, in the form of a patch, cream, gel, or lotion.

A wide variety of delivery systems for natural hormones are available. Prescription hormones are available in all the preceding forms, as well as sublinguals (dissolved under the tongue) and suppositories.

Transdermals—Creams and Gels   Creams are far more widely used in the United States than gels, but gels are slowly gaining ground and have been used in Europe for many years.

Both creams and gels are applied to parts of your body where the capillaries are near the surface of your skin and the product can be easily absorbed: your inner wrists, inner arms, face, stomach, breasts, neck, and palms. Some women feel comfortable rubbing a cream into their skin, but others find it messy or have a hard time accepting that they can get an accurate dose with this method (although they can). Typical dosages are ⅛ teaspoon or ½ teaspoon of the cream twice a day. You simply measure it into a kitchen measuring spoon, and eventually you can gauge how much to take without the spoon. Some gels made by European companies come with an applicator that makes it easy to measure out an exact dose.

Many doctors recommend creams or gels as a first choice because they deliver the natural hormone directly to your bloodstream. They are absorbed through the skin, so they bypass *first-pass elimination* by your liver. The liver breaks down hormones and works to eliminate them from your system. Usually, less than 10 percent of the original dosage is left after a hormone has passed through the liver. For this reason, oral dosages of hormones are considerably higher than dosages in creams or suppositories. When liver damage is associated with standard HRT, it is the result of the liver having to process and eliminate so many extra hormones.

Dr. Christiane Northrup, a well-known proponent of natural hormones, prefers creams because "absorption is very superior; however, there are many people who feel more comfortable with a pill, given our society."

Transdermals—Patches   Several proprietary (owned or patented exclusively by one drug company) natural estrogen patches are now on the market: Estraderm, Climera, and Vivelle.

Like creams and gels, the hormones in these patches are delivered through the skin. But patches can irritate your skin, and many women don't like the way the patch feels (it's usually worn on the buttocks). Additionally, the adhesive backing on the patches contains chemicals that can leach into your bloodstream along with the hormones. Patches probably don't present a huge risk, but all things considered—including that you can individualize the dose more easily with creams or gels—the latter are preferable.

Oral   Natural hormones can be produced as capsules, tablets, drops, or sublinguals—that is, small pills that dissolve under your tongue. Because progesterone's molecular structure is such that it is difficult to formulate in pill form, it must be first *micronized*— that is, broken down into very small particles. The particles are suspended in an oil base, which is then compounded into a form that can be taken orally. It's important to make sure that the oral progesterone you take has been formulated in this way. If you have gastrointestinal problems or liver problems, however, you should use creams or gels.

Micronized oral hormones are not absorbed quite as quickly as creams and gels, but they have two advantages. First, the dose can be measured very accurately. Second, American women are accustomed to taking pills and on some level "trust" them more than creams. If it's going to be easier to remember to take a pill or drops than to rub cream on your arms, an oral delivery system might be best for you.

Dr. Carolyn Shaak of WomenWell in Needham, Massachusetts, believes that the creams are a more "natural" delivery system than pills. Your ovaries secrete small amounts of hormones continuously throughout the day and night into a bed of blood vessels, and therefore natural hormones should be delivered directly into the bloodstream in their bio-identical form. She also believes that hormone levels cannot be kept as stable with oral delivery systems. When using a cream through the skin, your body fat acts as a storage depot for timed release of the hormones into your bloodstream, so hormone levels do not peak or fall to the degree that they would with pills. I urge you to try the creams first, as they are in general a more effective and safer delivery system.

Vaginal Suppositories   Since the 1940s, natural progesterone has been used in Europe in suppository form to treat PMS and menopausal symptoms. In the United States there is some resistance to using suppositories; consequently, this has not been a particularly popular delivery method. However, before the invention of micronized progesterone, progesterone in suppository form had been used for at least twenty-five years in the United States to treat PMS.

There are several good reasons for considering suppositories for HRT, however. Like transdermals, suppositories deliver hormones directly to the bloodstream, bypassing the liver and reducing the risk of liver damage. If you can't take the naturals orally because of gastrointestinal or liver problems, and you are uncomfortable using creams or gels, suppositories are a good choice. They come in a precise dosage, which is reassuring to women who do not like measuring out creams.

Suppositories are formulated in either a polyethylene glycol (PEG) base or a cocoa butter base. The PEG-based product delivers hormones to your bloodstream more completely and consistently than the cocoa butter–based product, but for many symptoms, the cocoa butter suppository works just fine.

One final note about suppositories: Make sure they are dissolving properly. If your suppository never fully dissolves, it's not delivering the correct dosage of hormones, and you may need to change brands.

What's a compounding pharmacy?

In the days before chain drugstores, pharmacists mixed—or *compounded*—drugs by hand. Chain drugstores sell only preformulated products, so the modern druggist's role has mostly been reduced to one of counting and bottling pills. Lately, however, compounding pharmacies have enjoyed a resurgence. Unlike the chains, they can customize prescriptions for the individual patient, fine-tuning a formula over weeks or months.

When your doctor or nurse practitioner orders natural hormones from a compounding pharmacy, he or she is giving the pharmacist a recipe designed specifically for you. Natural hormone products manufactured by companies such as Pharmacia Upjohn are similar to compounded products, but they have additives such as binders, fillers, or adhesives. Drugs from compounding pharmacies are free of these additives. For this reason, and because compounded naturals can be formulated to your specific needs, many physicians prefer them to the brand-name natural hormones.

You will want to choose a compounder with experience with natural hormones. Individualizing natural hormones requires precise measurements and skill in handling. Some of the larger pharmacies have twenty years' experience, have established large mail-order businesses, and work with doctors in all parts of the United States. If your doctor is already using natural hormones, he or she will almost certainly have established a ongoing relationship with a compounding pharmacist. Therefore, it is frequently not necessary for a woman to look for both a doctor *and* a compounder to work with.

There are now about 1,500 compounding pharmacies in the

United States. For a complete list of them, call the International Academy of Compounding Pharmacists at 800-927-4227; see also the Resource section, page 165, where we provide a list of compounding pharmacies that specialize in natural hormones.

If I want to use an over-the-counter natural hormone, how do I choose among them?

Before buying any natural hormone product, you'll need to read Chapter 4, "Finding Your Hormonal Profile." The type and dose you should take depends on your symptoms and profile. A young woman who needs relief from PMS may take a different product and dose than a woman entering menopause.

Once you know your hormonal profile and understand the types of hormones that will work best for you, your choice will depend on the delivery system you want. The following sections describe the over-the-counter natural hormone products currently available. But be aware that the over-the-counter products are not for everyone—for more intractable symptoms they might not be adequate, and even with the over-the-counter products, I recommend you work with a doctor if possible.

Creams   My personal favorite of the over-the-counter creams is Pro-Gest. It's been in use since the 1970s with great success. Transitions for Health, the company that makes it, sells about ten thousand jars a month. Another good product is Kokoro Balance Cream.

When purchasing an over-the-counter cream, remember that so-called wild yam creams are not the same thing as bio-identical hormone creams synthesized from wild yam. Many of these products contain diosgenin, the substance from which natural progesterone is made. But your own body can't make progesterone from diosgenin, so these creams contain no available progesterone and will not work! Just to create more confusion, some creams have both diosgenin and progesterone (made from diosgenin), and some creams are called wild yam creams and *do* contain progesterone. The bottom line is to make sure that the cream contains actual progesterone.

The packaging will list the number of milligrams of progesterone per ounce that the cream contains. As of this writing, there are no over-the-counter creams available in the United States for other natural hormones, such as estradiol. Ostaderm contains a tri-est formula.

The following creams contain more than 400 milligrams of progesterone per ounce:

Pro-Gest

Kokoro Balance Cream

Bio-Balance

Progonol

Ostaderm

Pro-Alo

Phyto-Gest

Natra-Gest

Happy PMS

Equilibrium

Pro-G

ProBalance

The following creams, which contain 0 to 15 milligrams of progesterone per ounce, *do not significantly affect progesterone levels in the body.* However, they may contain herbal supplements that provide relief of symptoms.

Pro-Dermex

Endocreme

Life Changes

Progesterone-Plus

Novagest

YamCon

Born Again

PMS Formula

Menopause Form

Femarone

Nutri-Gest

Herbal Formulas (in Pill Form)   Remifemin is a formulation of the herb *black cohosh*, and has been in use in Europe for over forty years to treat both PMS and menopausal symptoms. Black cohosh contains compounds that act similarly to human estriol in your body. Because no other herbal product has been so widely tested, I recommend Remifemin. It is a very effective product, but if you begin using it, be patient. Herbs are slower-acting than natural hormones, and so it will take a few weeks for you to begin to feel a change in your system. Remifemin is also used in conjunction with progesterone for a combination of hormone balancing and faster relief from symptoms. It's important to note that Remifemin is safe for women who have breast cancer or are at high risk for it.

If you can't find Remifemin, which is now available in most

health food stores, two other similar herbal products are Meno-Fem and Vitanica Women's Phase II. New to the marketplace as of 1998 is tablet-form Promensil, manufactured by Novogen Limited, an Australian company. Promensil provides 40 milligrams of phytoestrogen isoflavones extracted from red clover, which, according to the company's literature, contains four important isoflavones, as opposed to soy, which only contains two. As the packaging says: "The body converts phytoestrogen into phenolic estrogen, a form it can use to maintain estrogen supplies during midlife, when levels of ovarian estrogen decline." Several trials have been done on the product, and others are currently underway at various universities in the United States. To date, the product has shown promise and has been endorsed by a number of well-known menopause specialists. In Australia, more than three hundred women have participated in trials; in 1997 the Australian Menopause Society Congress found that Promensil was not associated with the side effects that may occur from prescription synthetic estrogen. Since no other drug available over the counter provides these phytoestrogen isoflavones, Promensil might be worth discussing with your doctor.

How much do natural hormones cost?

Because natural hormones are individualized—that is, formulated to meet your exact needs—the prescriptions can vary from simple to complex, and prices can range from as little as $8 a month to as much as $100. In 1999, average prices for compounded natural hormones were as follows:

* A prescription of 3 percent progesterone cream (30 milligrams per gram, taken at a rate of 1 gram a day) costs about $20 a month. Oral progesterone costs about $35 a month.

* Tri-est cream (2.5 milligrams per gram, taken at a rate of 1 gram a day) costs about $40 a month. An oral dose of tri-est costs about $20 to $25 monthly.

To find out exactly how much it would cost to switch from your current HRT to the naturals, simply call one of the compounding pharmacies listed in the Resources section, tell them the brand and dose you are taking, and they'll give you the price of the equivalent natural hormone.

Will my insurance company pay for natural hormones?

Many health insurance companies cover naturals, but they tend to make it complicated. Typically, they offer coverage on a reimbursement basis, meaning you have to fill out a form, send it to the insurer, and then wait for a reimbursement check. Some insurers cover naturals only if a doctor insists on them. "I end up writing a lot of letters for medical necessity based on my conviction that this is a safer and more effective way, or that some women just don't tolerate the standard hormones," reports Jesse Lynn Hanley, M.D. For the most part, she says, "If people get hormones they either buy them directly from the pharmacy or they pay at my office."

Compounding pharmacies have their own reasons for being reluctant to deal with insurance companies. The formula that insurers use to reimburse pharmacies is geared to drugs that have a single main ingredient. For mixtures such as tri-est, which contains three types of estrogen, compounding pharmacies get reimbursed only a fraction more than they spend on raw materials. It's a powerful disincentive to working with insurance companies.

The news is not all bleak, however. If you don't mind doing the paperwork, many insurance companies will reimburse you for natural hormones. And with every passing month, naturals are becoming more acceptable to mainstream medicine. One positive sign is that the National Institutes of Health recently established an office for alternative medicine. The more attention natural hormones receive from organizations such as this, the likelier it is that insurance companies will eventually loosen their restrictions on them.

If you're unhappy with your insurance company's policy on natural hormones, be sure to let them know. Write them a letter, and suggest that your physician do the same. When they hear from enough customers, they'll improve their coverage.

What does it mean to individualize hormones?

When your doctor tells you she is going to individualize your hormone treatment, she means that she will prescribe natural hormones formulated to meet your specific, individual needs. She'll need to test your hormone levels to establish a baseline level and find out exactly what these needs are; she should interview you at length about your symptoms. Your doctor may start you off on a precription natural hormone, or, depending on your symptoms and hormone levels, she may determine that an over-the-counter cream is adequate at first.

Individualized treatment depends on several things: the results of hormone level tests, your hormonal profile, and the way you respond to the hormones. A good physician will pay close attention to the feedback you give about side effects, energy level, and all the other facets of your well-being as the weeks progress. The tests you take are intended only as a starting point for your individualized treatment. Ultimately, your treatment will be determined by the way your body reacts to the hormones over the months and years. As you grow older and your body continues to change, your hormone treatment may change too.

This type of flexible treatment stands in stark contrast to the "one size fits all" approach of traditional HRT, which typically consists of Premarin or Premarin/Provera (or Prempro or Premphase). Even with natural hormones, discomfort can occur if you take too high a dose or are using the wrong combination for your particular symptoms. With individualized treatment, your hormone prescription can be fine-tuned until it provides maximum relief with minimum side effects.

If I use natural hormones, will my periods continue?

Using natural hormones will not cause your periods to cease. In fact, natural progesterone has been used in the United States and Europe for over fifty years to alleviate PMS symptoms and can be used to induce a period.

A natural progesterone product called Crinone 4% (Wyeth-Ayerst/Columbia Labs) recently received FDA approval and is now being used to promote menstrual cycles in female athletes suffering from secondary amenorrhea (absence of a monthly menstrual cycle). Although fewer than 3 percent of reproductive-age women have secondary amenorrhea, the rate is far higher among serious athletes—around 44 percent. So in this case, natural progesterone is used to reactivate periods.

If you are in perimenopause, taking natural progesterone can help alleviate the mood swings, weight gain, and other symptoms caused by the dominance of estrogen in your system during this time. The progesterone won't restore your normal periods if they have become infrequent and irregular, but it will stabilize your hormone levels and relieve menopause-like symptoms.

I'm on Premarin/Provera, but I want to quit taking them because of side effects. Before I switch to naturals, I'd like to get my hormone levels tested. Should I stop taking the Premarin/Provera altogether before I get tested? If so, for how long?

Many doctors consider it useful to test a woman's hormone levels before switching her from standard HRT to natural hormones. Women fluctuate greatly in their absorption rates of hormones when they are taken orally, as most HRT drugs are. Since side effects are partly a result of too much estrogen, it helps a doctor to know exactly how much estrogen is getting into your bloodstream from your current HRT. According to Dr. Carolyn Shaak, "Women who are taking other drugs that clear through the liver, or alcohol, or sedatives, may have surprisingly high levels of estrogen on Premarin . . . two to three times as high as they need to have."

Once the doctor knows where your hormone levels are, he or she can make a more accurate guess as to what's causing your discomfort and prescribe the naturals in dosages that will alleviate the problem. If you aren't having side effects but want to switch for health reasons, the tests will allow the doctor to match the dosage of natural hormones to the dosage in the synthetics that seems to be working for you.

Are natural hormones FDA-approved?

Much confusion exists in the medical community on this issue, and some doctors continue to believe that natural hormones lack FDA approval. In many cases, this stems from a lack of understanding of how the FDA approval system works.

Be assured that both natural hormones and the traditional HRT drugs (for example, Premarin/Provera) have the same level of FDA approval, and that natural hormones are made from FDA-approved substances. Per FDA guidelines, if natural hormones contain ingredients equivalent to already approved proprietary drugs, they can be prescribed by your doctor for the same indications.

Even though natural hormones are not specifically approved *drugs,* you must understand that it is not the FDA's mandate to find the best treatment for a problem. They merely decide whether the specific drugs submitted to them meet standards of safety and efficacy. An FDA-approved drug is not necessarily safer than any other remedy.

Certain natural hormone products are FDA-approved *drugs*— including Estrace and the patches Estraderm, Vivelle, and Climera, all of which are based on the plant-derived hormone estradiol. According to FDA guidelines, since natural estradiol prepared by a compounding pharmacist is identical to the estradiol in Estrace and other FDA-approved drugs, the compounded version is approved as well.

As of this writing, no drug company has applied for FDA approval of the plant-derived natural hormone estriol. However, this product—which exactly matches human estriol—has met the standards set by the U.S. Pharmacopeia, an organization that sets standards for all pharmaceuticals in the United States, and can be prescribed for you by your doctor.

I have a friend who is very happy with the Climera patch. How does a hormone patch work, and are there any risks involved?

Hormone patches deliver hormones to your bloodstream *transdermally*—that is, through the skin. The Climera patch (and the patches Estraderm and Vivelle) deliver natural, plant-derived estradiol. The adhesive, however, contains some chemical additives. Even if your friend loves her Climera patch and is experiencing no side effects from it, it might be worth her while to investigate other forms of natural hormone replacement. Climera is in the form of estradiol (E2), the strongest estrogen, and your friend might do just as well using a tri-est formula, which in the long run would be a much safer choice. It's important to always use estradiol *in combination with* progesterone, to provide hormonal balance and counteract any cancer risk from excess estrogen.

Some doctors prefer using tri-est (a combination of three estrogens), or estriol plus progesterone, as a first line of attack against menopausal symptoms. Other experts prescribe estradiol/

progesterone for relief of severe symptoms but suggest changing to tri-est/progesterone after six months, when symptoms have abated somewhat.

What about the brand-name oral natural estrogens such as Estrace and Estratest?

Estrace is an oral drug that is also derived from natural estradiol. It's been used in the United States since 1976. It should be taken in conjunction with progesterone, although unfortunately it is frequently prescribed singly. This brand-name estradiol is certainly preferable to Premarin—although the fact that it is a brand name doesn't impart any special effectiveness, and it has the same level of FDA approval as does the compounded natural estradiol.

Estratest is a combination of natural estradiol and methyltestosterone, a synthetic. Besides the fact that the testosterone is synthetic, I don't recommend it, as the amount of testosterone in this pill is too high and many women experience side effects such as acne, facial hair growth, and anxiety. In the long term, the methyltestosterone will also prove hard on your liver.

Recently Wyeth-Ayerst, maker of Premarin, introduced a generic estradiol tablet through one of its divisions. This shows an interest in protecting market share from all sides, and the use of this natural would be preferable to Premarin—but always in conjunction with progesterone.

Are there any brand-name natural progesterone products?

Two such products have come onto the market recently: Crinone and Prometrium.

Prometrium, manufactured by Schering-Plough and distributed in the United States by Solvay, is oral micronized natural progesterone in capsule form. The capsules contain peanut oil, so avoid this product if you're allergic to peanuts. A 100 mg. dose of Prometrium can make you sleepy, and it's recommended that you take it before bedtime. Most experts in the field of natural hormones prefer creams to pills, for reasons explained earlier (see page 96). Prometrium has not been FDA approved for treatment of menopausal symptoms, but many physicians prescribe it anyway.

Crinone 8% and Crinone 4%, manufactured by Wyeth-Ayerst/Columbia Labs, are natural progesterone gels packaged in a pre-filled vaginal applicator. Crinone 8% is used in fertility clinics to provide endometrial support for the growing fetus. Crinone 4% is used to restore periods to women who have ceased menstruating. Wyeth-Ayerst is also conducting clinical trials to see whether Crinone 4% is helpful in preventing hyperplasia (areas of excessive endometrial cells) in postmenopausal women who take estrogen. Clearly, the manufacturer is gearing up to market Crinone 4% as an HRT option.

As of this writing, the clinical trials on Crinone 4% for use in HRT have not been completed. Crinone gel is extremely expensive compared to other types of natural progesterone. The reason for this is that the method of application—the gel itself—is patented. It's specifically formulated to cling to the walls of the uterus because its main purpose is to make sure the endometrial lining stays put for fertility enhancement. This cling factor is a moot point for women who are seeking relief from menopause symptoms. In fact, it could be a detriment: The more the gel clings to your uterine walls, the less quickly the progesterone is absorbed into your bloodstream. Another concern is that your partner may absorb some of the progesterone during intercourse. Given all this, there seems to be little reason to use Crinone 4% in HRT.

When I asked my doctor about naturals, she suggested I try Ogen or Ortho-Est, which she said are plant-derived. Are they the same as naturals?

No. Many hormones are derived from plants, but that doesn't necessarily mean they are bio-identical. Ogen and Ortho-est fall into this category. They do come from plants, but their molecular structures are different from the structure of your body's hormones. Ogen and Ortho-Est do not exactly match the receptor sites on your cells the way bio-identical plant-derived hormones do. The word *bio-identical* is key—simply being plant-derived is not enough to make a product behave "naturally" in your body.

Are there side effects with naturals?

Side effects that occur with natural hormones are directly related to dose. When you first go to the doctor, you'll have your hormone levels tested and be given an initial prescription for estrogen and/or progesterone, and perhaps testosterone as well. The first prescription is a starting point only. The side effects of an incorrect dose of natural estrogen most commonly include water retention, weight gain, and breast tenderness. When the dose is adjusted, these symptoms abate.

Too much natural progesterone may result in mood changes, depression, and sleepiness. Again, the symptoms will usually vanish when the dose is fine-tuned. Similar side effects can occur with natural progesterone that is taken orally as opposed to in a cream, even if the dose is correct. The oral progesterone Prometrium, for example, comes in doses of 100 or 200 milligrams. Within four hours after taking Prometrium, your progesterone levels can shoot up to twice what they ever were during a normal menstrual period. This can result in drowsiness or mood swings. The problem isn't that 100 milligrams is too much—over the course of twenty-four hours, it's usually OK. It's just that your body fares better with smaller doses spread out over the day. Using a cream in the morning and at night delivers the progesterone to your bloodstream at a steadier rate, diminishing the chance of side effects. If you do choose Prometrium or another oral progesterone, take the pill at night so you can sleep through the side effects.

Too high a dose of natural testosterone can result in aggression, anxiety, acne, and growth of facial hair.

Very rarely, women will have side effects from the cream base itself—a redness or slight allergic reaction at the site where the cream was applied.

Will natural hormones make me gain weight as Premarin does?

The bloating and weight gain associated with Premarin result from too much estrogen in your system. Excess estrogen causes water retention. The type of estrogen doesn't matter—it can be produced by your body or introduced in the form of natural or synthetic hormones. For example, during PMS your body can produce excess estrogen, which causes the familiar bloating and swollen, sore breasts. During perimenopause, your body may become *estrogen dominant*—that is, it may accumulate an excess of estrogen relative to progesterone—which in turn can cause bloating and weight gain. HRT drugs such as Premarin, and natural estrogen in too strong a dose, will also increase your weight.

By taking naturals instead of Premarin you can avoid the weight gain problem for two reasons. First, with the naturals you can individualize your prescription. The amount of estrogen you take will be based upon your specific requirements, as determined by hormone level tests. Premarin is basically a "one size fits all" drug. Adjusting the dose is more difficult, and excess estrogen unbalanced by progesterone can cause weight gain.

The second reason you're not likely to gain weight on naturals is that the typical protocol includes progesterone along with the natural estrogen. Progesterone works to balance out the bloating effects of estrogen and actually helps the body eliminate fat.

Will taking natural hormones help normalize my sleep patterns?

Insomnia is a typical symptom of menopause. Its causes are not yet fully understood; while most people agree that hormones affect sleep, we know little about *how* they affect it. Certainly women who suffer from night sweats have a hard time sleeping soundly, but other women also find their sleep patterns disrupted during menopause.

One thing experts do seem to agree on is that natural progesterone taken just before bed helps women sleep better. Increased drowsiness is one of the few side effects of progesterone, and it can be overcome by dividing up your dose (of cream) and taking it two times a day. If you want the soporific effect, you can purposely take a larger portion at bedtime. If you're taking oral progesterone, it's recommended that you take it at nighttime because the dose is likely to make you sleepy and perhaps a little moody. Ingesting it before bed allows you to sleep though the moodiness and get a good night's rest.

If you get night sweats, a combination of estrogen (to alleviate the sweats) and progesterone may offer the most relief.

Chapter Seven

PMS, HORMONE IMBALANCE, AND NATURAL HORMONES

It is commonly assumed that natural hormone replacement is only an option for older women, but whether you're dealing with PMS or a more serious hormonal imbalance problem—such as endometriosis or fibrocystic breasts—natural hormones should be the first line of defense. Natural progesterone can be especially useful for PMS, and by dealing with the issue of hormone balance issues early on, you can prevent the need for more extreme measures, such as a hysterectomy, and save yourself a lot of unnecessary suffering.

Does progesterone help alleviate PMS?

Since the 1950s, European doctors have used progesterone to treat symptoms of PMS. In the United States, progress was much slower in this regard—in fact, PMS was not even recognized as a legitimate syndrome until the 1970s. It wasn't until about that time that progesterone was made available to women in this country. The British physician who pioneered the use of progesterone to combat PMS, Dr. Katherina Dalton, is the same one who battled to have PMS recognized as a physiological rather than a mental condition. In the 1940s Dr. Dalton began treating PMS with progesterone in suppository form. She has treated more than thirty thousand women successfully, reporting that progesterone is extremely safe and effective in alleviating PMS. In 1977, she published the results of her treatment in a book titled *Premenstrual Syndrome and Progesterone Therapy*.

The underlying causes of PMS can vary from woman to woman and may be triggered by factors other than hormone imbalance. However, balancing hormones should be the key component of any PMS treatment, and here progesterone is very effective, particularly for reducing anxiety and mood swings.

Remifemin, an herbal remedy based on black cohosh and distributed in this country by Enzymatic Therapy, can also be very effective for PMS. It works by balancing your estrogen levels, raising or lowering them as needed. First developed in Germany, it is the number one bestselling product for PMS and menopause in that country.

My periods can be very irregular. Can naturals help me?

Until about age 40, the majority of women have regular periods (28- to 30-day cycles). Then, heading toward menopause, a woman's periods can begin to get irregular. Sometimes irregular periods are caused by a lack of ovulation or because of ovarian cysts. It is standard treatment to prescribe a progestin (either Provera or a birth control pill) for this condition. Natural progesterone can do a better job, without the potential side effects of the progestins. Dr. John Lee suggests you use the smallest dose of progesterone cream at first to support your regular monthly cycling down of progesterone.

I have excessive bleeding and my doctor has prescribed Provera. Will this help? Can I take natural progesterone instead?

When women—especially those in perimenopause—have excessive menstrual bleeding, it's often due to estrogen dominance. (Estrogen dominance refers to the *ratio* of estrogen to progesterone, not the overall levels of each hormone.) Your doctor has prescribed the progestin Provera to restore some balance to your system and limit the effects of the estrogen. Natural progesterone will accomplish the same thing.

Women who have excessive bleeding are also frequently prescribed birth control pills (which also contain synthetic progestin), which can exacerbate the problem. Women with this problem are in the greatest danger of being hysterectomized. Resist this suggestion to just "take it out" to solve the problem.

For more information on hysterectomies, see the Bibliography for suggested reading.

I have fibrocystic breasts. Can natural hormones help me?

Too many women suffer from this painful condition, which is commonly the result of estrogen dominance. You can relieve your painful, lumpy breasts by using progesterone cream. You can rub it right on your breasts, which can resolve the problem more quickly. Also follow the dietary recommendations for PMS (see Chapter 3, page 41), particularly abstinence from coffee.

I have fibroids. My doctor has recommended a hysterectomy. A friend said she eliminated her fibroids by taking progesterone. Is this possible?

You should definitely first try progesterone. Fibroids develop over time and when they cause excessive bleeding, a woman is at great risk for a hysterectomy. After menopause, fibroids almost always shrink, but before that time they can be a source of discomfort for many women. Progesterone can be used to shrink the fibroids, but you must be patient. Give it at least a few months, as the fibroid took some time to grow to a size that came to cause your problems. If removal of the fibroids seems necessary before resorting to a hysterectomy, investigate laser surgery first, which removes the fibroids without removing the uterus.

Chapter Eight

FERTILITY, BIRTH CONTROL PILLS, AND NATURAL HORMONES

The synthesis of natural progesterone in the 1940s ultimately led to the development of birth control pills and fertility treatments. Recently gynecologists have begun advising women in their thirties and forties to take birth control pills for noncontraceptive concerns, such as PMS and protection against endometrial and ovarian cancer. However, these same benefits can be gained from natural hormones, with none of the risks and side effects of birth control pills.

I'm trying to get pregnant, and I've heard that fertility clinics use natural progesterone as part of their treatment plan. Can I do it myself with progesterone cream?

Natural progesterone is used in some fertility clinics to increase the likelihood that a fertilized egg will survive. While I hesitate to recommend that a woman embark on a home-grown fertility plan without being monitored by a physician, I am aware that some women use progesterone cream on their own for this purpose. In his monthly newsletter, progesterone expert Dr. John Lee laid down the following guidelines for women who want to use progesterone cream as a fertility aid.

First, be sure you are using a pure, natural progesterone cream that has no other ingredients. *Do not use any synthetic proges-*

tins—they are not the same as progesterone and can cause birth defects. Dr. Lee advises women to use the cream after ovulation, and to continue using 30 milligrams twice daily if you become pregnant. Do not suddenly stop using the cream, as this may trigger a miscarriage. If you don't get pregnant, stop using the cream at the onset of your period. Wait until just after ovulation to use the cream again.

My own recommendation is to seek the counsel of your doctor before using progesterone cream for fertility purposes.

I'm 35 and still get PMS like a 14-year-old. I use a diaphragm for birth control. If I take natural progesterone to control my PMS, will it make me more fertile?

The role of natural progesterone in fertility treatments is to increase the likelihood that a fertilized egg will survive in the uterus. The protocol I recommend for PMS involves using progesterone cream in the same doses, or greater, as those Dr. Lee recommends using for fertility (see previous question), and during roughly the same time in your cycle. So taking the cream for PMS may increase the likelihood that a fertilized egg will survive. If you suddenly stop taking the progesterone, it might cause a miscarriage, but that would be an extremely unreliable form of birth control! My advice: If you take progesterone for PMS, use the diaphragm religiously, and if you're especially concerned about not getting pregnant, refrain from sex on the days, before, during, and immediately after ovulation.

My sister had horrible postpartum depression. Can I take natural hormones after I deliver my baby to avoid this condition?

The latest method for treating postpartum depression is to use natural progesterone. You'll recall that when you're not pregnant, your ovaries produce most of the progesterone in your body. The output is cyclical, ranging from 2 to 3 milligrams a day to a peak of perhaps 30 milligrams a day. When you're in your third trimester, your placenta produces 350 to 400 milligrams of progesterone a day, while your ovaries produce none.

After you give birth, the placenta is no longer there to produce progesterone. Your ovaries have not yet begun to produce it, so your progesterone levels plummet. It seems likely that there is a connection between this sudden drop in progesterone and postpartum blues. Consequently, some doctors have begun treating the condition with natural progesterone. While there is little track record for this use of the hormone, two experts in the field recommend it.

"Anybody who is at risk for postpartum depression should be taking natural progesterone the minute the baby is born," states Dr. Christiane Northrup in an interview for *International Journal of Pharmaceutical Compounding* (January/February 1998). "Full-blown postpartum depression is completely unrecognized and undertreated. . . . [If someone] has had postpartum depression before, then there is a good reason for using progesterone."

Dr. John Lee concurs, and advises women to "measure progesterone levels a day or two after childbirth and, if found to be low, progesterone could be promptly supplemented. It is possible that this simple and safe therapy could make postpartum depression much easier to treat."

Do birth control pills "mask" symptoms of perimenopause?

Birth control pills shut down the natural production of estrogen and progesterone and replace them with a low, steady supply of estrogen and synthetic progestins. By doing so, they regulate your menstrual cycles and the amount of hormones circulating through your body. This can alleviate many of the symptoms of perimenopause, including mood swings, insomnia, hot flashes, PMS, night sweats, and even heart palpitations. In essence, then, birth control pills do mask the symptoms of perimenopause. In fact, gynecologists have begun to "treat" perimenopause with birth control pills.

> *When I told my gynecologist I was beginning to feel as if I'm in perimenopause, he prescribed the contraceptive pill Loestrin to keep my bones strong and reduce my mood swings. I'm not even in a relationship! Does this make sense?*

Because it regulates the hormones in your body, the Pill can mitigate symptoms of perimenopause (see page 123). There are plenty of caveats, however. Although a recent study supported by drug companies supposedly laid to rest women's fears of the long-term risks of birth control pills for breast cancer, cervical cancer, and stroke, a group of doctors called the Cancer Prevention Coalition have disputed the claims of the study and draw attention to the sharp rise in estrogen-dependent breast cancers since the advent of the Pill. Physicians generally agree that the Pill is not appropriate for women who smoke or are predisposed to heart disease or high blood pressure. Some doctors go further, recommending that women with high cholesterol or diabetes stay away from the Pill. If you have ever had a blood clot you should definitely avoid the Pill, as it increases the likelihood of a second clot.

Some women may feel only the Pill can meet their contraceptive needs, but if you're not in a relationship, you can get the same benefits of symptom relief and bone protection, and even more, from natural hormones.

> *I'm 42 and have been on birth control pills for five years. I'd like to get off, but my gynecologist told me I should keep taking them because they protect against endometrial and ovarian cancer. Is he right? What are the natural hormone alternatives to the Pill in terms of cancer protection?*

Most women should never take the Pill. The question of whether to use the Pill for cancer protection is more complicated than it first seems. After all, the Pill does carry a slightly increased risk of breast cancer for all women who take it. As for protection against endometrial cancer, unless there is reason to believe you are at high risk, there is no reason to "risk" continued use of the Pill. Most of the conditions that would put you at high risk for endometrial cancer are related to estrogen dominance, which caused endometrial cancer in the early users of unopposed Premarin and prompted drug manufacturers to add a synthetic progestin (Provera) to oppose the estrogen. If you are concerned about endometrial cancer risk, a hormone level test will give you a good idea of the ratio between your estrogen and progesterone and whether you're estrogen dominant. If you are, natural progesterone will restore your hormone balance and provide the same cancer protection as birth control pills.

I'm 44 and am taking birth control pills, but I'm curious as to whether I'm in perimenopause. Can I get my hormone levels tested even though I'm on the Pill?

No. According to Dr. Carolyn V. Shaak, an expert in the field of natural hormones, a woman should be off birth control pills for at least six weeks before getting her hormone levels tested. If you do go off the Pill in order to get your hormone levels tested, be sure to use an alternate method of birth control.

Chapter Nine

PERIMENOPAUSE AND NATURAL HORMONES

*U*ntil recently, women in perimenopause suffering such symptoms as fatigue, anxiety, and weight gain got little attention from their doctors. Fortunately, the distress caused by the extreme hormonal shiftings of perimenopause can be well managed with changes in diet, nutritional supplements, and natural hormones.

> *I'm 46. About a year ago I noticed a drastic change in my emotions—I cry at the least provocation. My doctor suggested Prozac, but that seems extreme. Can I treat my blues with natural hormones?*

At age 46 you could be entering perimenopause, which brings a slew of changes to your hormonal makeup. It's not uncommon for doctors to misdiagnose the symptoms of perimenopause, which can include depression. Physicians often prescribe antidepressants such as Prozac to give women some relief from perimenopausal depression, but you're right—it may not be necessary to go to such extremes.

Why do women in perimenopause experience depression and emotional sensitivity? One of the key factors is that at this time in your life, your ovaries slow down their production of progesterone. The balance you've maintained all your adult life—the particular ratios of progesterone to estrogen—is thrown off, and you body may enter a phase of estrogen dominance. During this time, your estrogen levels can fluctuate dramatically, while your output of progesterone stays low. Every woman reacts to estrogen dominance differently, but typical symptoms include mood swings, depression, fatigue, irritability, inability to handle stress, headaches, low sex drive, water retention, and weight gain.

The first line of attack against these symptoms should be to reestablish your hormonal balance and eat a healthier diet. See whether your outlook improves after a few months of the new regimen, and then decide whether you need Prozac. Perhaps you are going through a psychological crisis that is causing you to cry easily; perhaps you do need antidepressants (or for that matter, a therapist). In fact, it's wise to consult a therapist before taking an antidepressant because he or she can work with you to determine the best course of treatment. But even if you are going through a psychological crisis, a hormonal imbalance could be exacerbating your moodiness. By yourself, you might not be able to figure out whether your depression is due to a psychological crisis, perimenopause, or both. Whatever the case, it makes sense to tackle any hormonal imbalance before you decide to take drugs.

In Chapter 4, "Finding Your Hormonal Profile," you can read about the symptoms associated with perimenopause. This chapter also tells what you can do to combat those symptoms, such as eating a healthy diet; getting exercise; taking vitamin, mineral, and herbal supplements; and in some cases using natural hormone therapy. Remifemin and Pro-Gest (or other equivalent creams such as Kokoro Balance Creme) are good options. Also, consider getting your hormone levels tested, and if warranted try a natural progesterone cream. It's very likely that these measures will put an end to your crying jags.

If your doctor isn't knowledgeable about hormone balancing or seems resistant to your questions, seek the advice of a different doctor. The section titled "How to Work with a Doctor" in Chapter 2 will give you some guidelines. Also, NWI can provide you with a listing of practitioners in your local area who work with natural hormones.

I'm in perimenopause and have started to suffer from severe
headaches and anxiety attacks. Can natural hormones help me?

Headaches and anxiety attacks are common symptoms of perimenopause. They can be brought on by estrogen dominance—
that is, fluctuating levels of estrogen insufficiently balanced by progesterone. Anxiety is just one of several emotions that can be in-
tensified by estrogen dominance.

Estrogen dominance also causes blood vessels to dilate more
easily; this, in combination with the water-retention effects of estrogen, can lead to migraine headaches. Many women suffer from
migraines just prior to getting their periods, when estrogen is at
its peak in their system. The same principle is at work when you
get headaches due to your estrogen levels rising suddenly in perimenopause. Fortunately, you can take natural progesterone to balance the effects of estrogen, and this should provide some
headache relief. Once you get your hormone levels tested, you
should be able to tell how much hormone replacement you need
to rebalance your system.

It also may be possible for you to alleviate some of your symptoms by changing your diet. Caffeine is a stimulant and can cause
anxiety—so, difficult as it may be, try going without coffee for a
few weeks. If your periods are no longer regular, it may be worth
your while to cut out the caffeine entirely for a month and see if
there is any improvement in your mood.

In addition to caffeine, there are other "feel-bad" foods you
ought to avoid: sugar, salt, alcohol, diet sodas, and chocolate and
cocoa (which contain caffeine and refined sugar). These foods are
known to aggravate hormonal imbalance symptoms, and some of
them are harmful to your body in other ways. You may eventually
be able to add some back into your diet in moderation, but if you
drastically limit them for a few weeks you'll be able to gauge the
effect they are having on your anxiety and headaches.

I seem to be losing my sex drive. Help!

Beginning in perimenopause and sometimes continuing for the rest of their lives, some women experience a decline in sex drive. For many years this decline was attributed to decreasing estrogen levels. It now seems likely that two other hormones—progesterone and testosterone—may play a more important role.

Dr. John Lee has probably done more extensive research in this area than anyone else to date, having treated women for menopausal complaints for more than thirty years. In his book *What Your Doctor May Not Tell You About Menopause*, Dr. Lee recounted his observations about the impact of estrogen replacement alone, and estrogen with progesterone, on the libido of his patients.

As his patients approached midlife, Dr. Lee noticed that some were feeling more sexually active than they had before, while others were losing their appetite for sex. He became convinced that those with diminishing sex drive were experiencing estrogen dominance: "The women losing interest in sex had water retention; fibrocystic breasts; depression; dry, wrinkling skin; and irregular, sometimes heavy periods . . . these signs and symptoms were indicative of a progesterone deficiency caused by a failure to ovulate while estrogen continued to be produced, which is to say loss of sex drive correlates with progesterone deficiency, not estrogen deficiency." Dr. Lee encountered many patients who were already taking estrogen and still complained of low libido. When he treated these women with 20–30 milligrams of progesterone a day, in a cream format, their sex drive improved.

An important aspect of Dr. Lee's decades-long informal survey is that *too much progesterone decreases libido rather than increasing it*. Balancing the estrogen and progesterone levels in your body is crucial. Taking too much progesterone will be counterproductive. Dr. Lee explains, "Many physicians, for reasons I do not understand, opt for doses 10 to 20 times higher [than 30 milligrams]. When they report that they do not see a resurgence of sex drive as I have found in my patients, it is not a surprise to me."

Testosterone has also been shown to improve libido. If you and your doctor are considering testosterone replacement, be sure to test your levels at the appropriate time of day (see Chapter 2, page 22). Too much testosterone can have unpleasant side effects, such as aggression, anxiety, excess facial hair, and acne. The side effects of too much progesterone (sleepiness, moodiness) can be controlled by reducing the dose.

I'm in perimenopause and my doctor gave me Estrace. It didn't help at all—in fact, it made me feel worse. Why is that?

This is a common occurrence for women in perimenopause. During this time, your estrogen levels can be fluctuating dramatically in relation to your progesterone, and adding estrogen can actually make you feel much worse and complicate your symptoms of estrogen dominance. Your best choice would be a progesterone cream, which would balance your spiking estrogen levels. As progesterone is a precursor hormone, your body could convert the progesterone to estrogen, if there is a need for it.

Chapter Ten

MENOPAUSE AND NATURAL HORMONES

*B*y the time a woman reaches menopause she is almost certainly aware of the controversy surrounding standard hormone replacement therapy drugs, principally Premarin and Provera. Unfortunately, these synthetic drugs, with their significant side effects and risk factors, have become synonymous with estrogen and progesterone, thereby confusing women who are concerned, for example, about increased risk of breast cancer. Many women who could benefit from hormone replacement choose to forgo it rather than put themselves at risk. They need to know that natural hormones are a far better and safer solution and that they can use the naturals to reap many health benefits without undue concern.

Since menopause began, I could swear my brain cells are dying off. I'm getting really scattered, and it's beginning to frighten me. What's going on, and can natural hormones help?

There is debate among experts about exactly why some menopausal women suffer from a lack of focus and mental clarity. The makers of standard HRT drugs (Premarin and others), as well as numerous physicians, claim that estrogen replacement can sharpen brain function. Other experts insist that replacing progesterone, not estrogen, is key to maintaining mental acuity after menopause.

The fact is, more research will need to be done before we know exactly how estrogen and/or progesterone affect the brain. We do know that estrogen plays an important role in brain function by promoting the production of an enzyme that helps keep connections between brain cells healthy. A 1994 study published in *Obstetrics and Gynecology* found that estrogen helped maintain verbal learning and enhanced a woman's ability to learn new information after menopause. It's known that estrogen affects nearly every part of your brain, including memory, ability to focus, attention span, and mental acuity. Therefore, it is widely assumed that estrogen replacement will help in these areas during and after menopause.

But there is another side to the story, explained by Dr. John Lee in *What Your Doctor May Not Tell You About Menopause*. According to Dr. Lee, estrogen dominance, which some women experience in menopause, suppresses thyroid function. "When thyroid function is low," writes Dr. Lee, "cellular oxygen is low. . . . Thus estrogen-induced thyroid interference contributes to less-than-optimal brain function." The reasoning is that low cell oxygen impedes brain function. Dr. Lee claims to have successfully treated many "scattered" women with progesterone, including women who were already taking estrogen replacement but were unsatisfied with the results.

I entered menopause about two years ago, and my mood swings are driving me (and my family) crazy. Will natural hormones help stabilize my emotions?

The mood swings that torment so many women at menopause are not unlike those you might have experienced when you were pregnant, or the postpartum blues that might have set in after you gave birth. These mood swings were primarily due to shifting hormones. New mothers eventually regain hormonal balance, but women in menopause could continue having mood swings for a long time unless they intervene with some form of hormone replenishment. Many women complain that they no longer feel like themselves; they are depressed, weepy, touchy, and anxiety-ridden.

Months go by and nothing changes. For some, the situation drags on for years.

Because "the change" is a significant milestone in a woman's life, many people, including physicians, once claimed these problems were purely psychological. Now, however, there is ample evidence to show that hormonal imbalance is to blame for the mood swings of menopause. And yes, natural hormones do help many women get their emotions back to normal.

Here's how the hormones estrogen and progesterone affect your mood. When you exercise or experience something pleasurable, your brain produces higher levels of noradrenaline, a substance that, simply put, makes you feel good. Noradrenaline, in turn, is kept in check by an enzyme called MAO (monoamine oxidase). Estrogen inhibits MAO—that is, it prevents your body from producing too much of it. When estrogen levels drop, MAO levels rise and do too good a job of suppressing noradrenaline. As a result, you feel depressed. For this reason, replacing estrogen may help elevate your mood.

The role of progesterone in the brain is not well understood, but it has earned the nickname "the feel-good hormone" because of its positive effect on mood. We do know that there is twenty times more progesterone in your brain cells than in your bloodstream, which points to progesterone playing a very important role in your brain function and emotions. Natural hormone therapy stresses balancing estrogen and progesterone, so if you decide to try the natural, you will reap the benefits of both hormones.

My hot flashes have become a nonstop source of embarrassment to me. Can natural hormones provide some relief?

Hot flashes are the most widely recognized symptoms of menopause. Those who haven't experienced them may joke about the affliction, but anyone who has suffered through hot flashes knows how debilitating they can be. In addition to the discomfort, it's certainly awkward being the one person who is always asking that a window be opened or the air conditioner cranked up.

Natural hormones can mitigate hot flashes just as well as standard HRT drugs such as Premarin, and are a safer choice. Some women can control hot flashes using just progesterone, but others with severe symptoms might need a combination estrogen/progesterone. If your hot flashes are mild, you might consider phytoestrogen products such as Remifemin or Promensil (see the Resources section, page 165). Most important, when you begin getting hot flashes, you should work on all fronts to stabilize your hormones by improving your diet and adding nutritional supplements and exercise. Your hot flashes can be a wake-up call that puts you on a road to having the best health of your life.

I'm experiencing a lot of vaginal dryness since I stopped my periods. It's seriously interfering with my sex life. Can hormones help?

Next to hot flashes, vaginal dryness and thinning of the vaginal wall are the most common symptoms of menopause. They can lead to *vaginal atrophy*, a shortening and narrowing of the vaginal cavity. These conditions combined can also contribute to pain during intercourse.

There is a two-pronged approach to these symptoms. First, using natural estrogen and progesterone will improve this condition over time, depending on the woman and the severity of the condition. If you do not have other severe menopausal symptoms, a transdermal natural progesterone cream may be all you need. The next step up would be natural estrogen/progesterone. In the meantime, you can also use a vaginal gel or cream containing natural estradiol or estriol. The typical protocol for a topical vaginal preparation is a small dose applied twice a week, three weeks a month.

I've been on Premarin/Provera for five years and I feel fine. Why should I switch to natural hormones?

Some women do feel fine on the Premarin/Provera program, and whenever you're comfortable with a product, it's hard to change. However, feeling fine now doesn't reduce the potential health risks associated with Premarin/Provera. There are hidden dangers.

With long-term use, Premarin/Provera may put women at risk for endometrial cancer, breast cancer, ovarian cancer, gallbladder disease, liver disease, and stroke. A recent study in the *Journal of the American Chemical Society* reported finding a by-product of Premarin that damaged DNA in a way that could cause cancer.

We believe it's wiser to choose natural hormones. Because they match your own hormones exactly, they have fewer risks than Premarin and other synthetics. Natural hormones provide all the alleged benefits of Premarin/Provera—protection against osteoporosis and potential heart disease, and relief from menopausal symptoms.

How do I switch from Premarin/Provera (also Prempro and Premphase) to the naturals?

The answer is, very easily. A compounding pharmacist creates an equivalent dose of the naturals—tri-est, or bi-est, or estradiol, plus progesterone—and then you simply stop taking the Premarin/Provera and start taking the naturals.

If you've been enduring negative side effects from Premarin/Provera, you have two choices. Your side effects may be entirely due to your body's negative reaction to the synthetic hormones, in which case you can simply start with an equivalent dose of the naturals and see how you feel. Or you can start with a lower dose of the naturals, and your doctor can adjust the doses as necessary, based on your response. Many women get relief from side effects within a few days of making the switch, but you and your doctor may need to fine-tune the ratio of estrogen and progesterone until you are free of side effects and get a good amount of relief from menopausal symptoms as well.

If you are postmenopausal and taking Premarin/Provera to

guard against osteoporosis, please be sure to read the hormone profile for postmenopausal women in Chapter 4 (pages 56–58). You may need only progesterone and dietary supplements, along with a program of healthy diet and exercise, to protect yourself against bone loss. If you do need both estrogen and progesterone, you can use natural hormones instead of Premarin/Provera to get the same protection. You'll need to get your hormone levels tested to see which protocol is right for you. You will also find that you will no longer continue to bleed when you are taking naturals—a very important plus!

> *I hear that soy contains phytoestrogens. Can I control my menopausal symptoms by just eating lots of tofu?*

Probably not. Soy in the form of tofu does contain isoflavones, which are structurally similar to human estrogen. Adding it to your diet can have great benefits for cancer protection and can bring about some of the benefits touted for estrogen—such as lowering so-called bad cholesterol and improving brain function. Tofu is a staple in the Asian diet and may be responsible for lower cancer rates in those cultures and also for the fact that Asian women have a much lower incidence of menopausal symptoms. Having it in your diet from a very young age could conceivably protect you from menopausal symptoms in later life. But just adding it to your diet at the onset of menopausal symptoms is unlikely to control them sufficiently. A recent study at the Bowman-Gray School of Medicine that tested soy protein isolates in menopausal women found that although the intensity of the participants' hot flashes was reduced, the number of hot flashes was not.

A leading researcher in the field, David Zava, Ph.D., warns that it makes a difference what *kind* of soy you eat. "There are an enormous number of toxins (*antinutrients*) in unfermented soy. . . . If you are not allergic to soyfoods, eat them primarily as fermented soy products, which includes miso and tempeh." According to Dr.

Zava, unfermented soyfoods such as tofu should be eaten with sea vegetables or fish to counteract the antinutrients.

In sum, adding soy to your diet is undoubtedly good for your overall health, but eating large amounts of it to cure your change-of-life symptoms is unlikely to do much good. A new product, Revival, contains 20 grams of protein and 160 milligrams of soy estrogens. (A typical serving of tofu or soybeans contains 20 grams of protein and only about 30 milligrams of soy estrogens.) Taking this product with its higher amount of soy estrogens may work in controlling your symptoms; talk to your doctor about it.

I've heard about taking black cohosh for menopausal symptoms. Is this a natural hormone?

Black cohosh is not a natural hormone. It is an herb that contains compounds that have an estrogenic effect in your body—they act similarly to human estriol. Their main function is to stabilize your own hormones; if your body needs more estrogen, the compounds enhance the effects of your body's own estrogen. If your body has too much estrogen, the compounds inhibit the effects of your own estrogen.

The most widely tested form of black cohosh is a product called Remifemin, distributed in the United States by Enzymatic Therapy and sold as a dietary supplement. It has been the subject of extensive testing and has been used in Europe for more than forty years as a remedy for PMS and menopausal symptoms. Remifemin provides all the symptom relief some women need; others find it helpful when used in conjunction with natural progesterone. Because it has been proven not to stimulate cell growth in the breast, Remifemin is especially beneficial to women who have breast cancer or are at risk for it and therefore must avoid estrogens.

Can traditional herbal remedies such as dong quai relieve my menopausal symptoms?

Depending on the severity of your symptoms, traditional herbal medicines may or may not be useful. Many women do find relief using the herbs listed here, some of which have been in use for hundreds of years. They are produced by a number of manufacturers. Reliable brands include Enzymatic Therapy, Gaia, Zand, Herb Pharm, Eclectic Institute, Naturally Vitamins, and Tyler Encapsulations. Herbal remedies can be purchased at pharmacies, health food stores, and some grocery stores.

Chaste tree berry helps balance estrogen and progesterone. It is slow-acting and its effects are felt after a few months of daily use. It's especially beneficial for women who go through early menopause, either naturally or due to hysterectomy.

Dong quai is a root that has been used for thousands of years in China to treat "women's complaints." It has an analgesic effect on the uterus and also has been shown to reduce bloating, lower blood pressure, and increase oxygen consumption in the liver. Results will become evident after about two weeks. Dong quai is often used in combination with other herbs.

Evening primrose oil, used to treat both PMS and menopausal symptoms, is a traditional Native American medicine. Recent studies indicate that evening primrose oil may help prevent hardening of the arteries, heart disease, and high blood pressure, in addition to its other benefits.

Gamma oryzanol is an extract of rice bran oil. A 1984 study in Japan tested the product's efficacy for menopausal symptoms, and results were positive: Women who took 300 milligrams per day reported an 85 percent improvement in symptoms within two months. Meno-Fem by Prevail is a good source of gamma oryzanol; Tyler Encapsulations also markets gamma oryzanol.

Ginseng contains plant hormones, essential fatty acids, antioxidants, minerals, and glycosides. It can be very helpful in alleviating menopausal symptoms, but like most herbal remedies, it takes about two weeks for the effects to become noticeable.

Licorice root helps support natural adrenal function and has been found to behave similarly to hormones produced by the adrenal glands. The adrenal glands produce a low level of sex hormones at midlife.

Wild yam is not the same thing as natural progesterone synthesized from wild yam. Still, it can be used to balance your own hormones. For thousands of years women have used wild yam to prevent miscarriage, ease menstrual cramps, and relieve menopausal symptoms. It's often included in combination herbal products for midlife women.

Vitamin E has been the subject of several studies that indicated it was helpful in alleviating hot flashes and night sweats. It has also been shown to have important benefits for women in the prevention of heart disease. It is best taken in combination with other vitamins, minerals, and antioxidants, as it isn't as effective on its own.

I'm 55 and feel fine. My doctor just prescribed Premarin/Provera because he says I have to protect myself against heart disease and osteoporosis. What should I do?

Let's take a close look at the merits of Premarin/Provera in protecting against heart disease and osteoporosis. As far as heart disease is concerned, the jury is still out. The 1995 PEPI study found that women using Premarin/Provera showed raised "good" cholesterol (HDL) levels and lowered "bad" cholesterol (LDL) levels. The study also found that the participants had reduced levels of fibrinogen, a blood clotting agent. The question is, do these findings automatically mean that Premarin prevents heart disease?

No, they don't. Plenty of drugs that lower cholesterol do not reduce the risk for heart disease, and some actually increase the risk. A diet that is lower in fat and cholesterol is generally seen as healthier for your heart, but that doesn't mean drugs that lower your cholesterol are necessarily going to protect you from heart disease.

The reduced levels of blood-clotting fibrinogen did not result in health benefits for any of the 975 women in the PEPI study. In fact, ten of them developed blood clots during the study, while none of the women in the placebo group developed clots—hardly a ringing endorsement for that "benefit" of Premarin/Provera.

As for osteoporosis, natural progesterone is more effective than Premarin/Provera at stopping bone loss and building new bone mass. Premarin and Premarin/Provera have been shown to slow the loss of bone but not to *build* bone, as progesterone does. (Testosterone has also been shown to build new bone.) Plus, in order to have the positive effect on your bones, you must take Premarin/Provera for a number of years. Unfortunately, the longer you take it, the more you put yourself at risk for breast and endometrial cancer.

Tell your doctor that you are not willing to take those risks when the benefits of Premarin/Provera are not completely certain. Instead, suggest that the two of you work out a plan for a healthy diet, exercise, and perhaps some natural progesterone if you're at risk for osteoporosis. Get tested first! Don't assume that just because you're 55 you have a propensity for brittle bones. The same goes for heart disease. If you are healthy and have no family history of heart disease, why take a potentially harmful synthetic hormone to guard against it?

Keep in mind that recent studies indicate that more than twenty-five million Americans, mostly women, are at risk for osteoporosis. The disease leads to numerous problems (such as spinal compression fractures and broken hips) that can make your final years very uncomfortable. If you get tested and learn that you are at risk for it, a good diet, exercise, and a natural hormone such as progesterone may make the difference between an active "golden age" and misery.

Some women do sail through menopause with little discomfort. However, don't be too quick to discount natural hormone replacement. It could be that you've learned to put up with mildly annoying symptoms because you're a tough-it-out type of person and you don't believe in complaining about a little insomnia here, a diminishing interest in sex, or a bit of middle-age spread. You just chalk it up to getting older. If this sounds like you, I think you'll be surprised by the hormone profile for menopause in Chapter 4 (page 53). You may have gotten used to certain changes in your body without realizing that they are caused by a hormonal imbalance. An individualized prescription for natural hormones, calibrated to give you exactly the amount your body needs, may make you feel altogether younger and more vital.

Of course, some women don't need any hormone replacement at all. Other women use natural hormones for their anti-aging properties, but this is a personal choice. Still others use hormone replacement during menopause, but don't choose to continue it in later years. By having your hormone levels tested, you'll be able to intelligently choose the option that is healthiest for you.

There is heart disease in my family. I have no real menopausal symptoms, but should I take estrogen for prevention?

You need to determine the most beneficial, least harmful program for a healthy heart. See page 139 for an explanation of why the findings concerning Premarin/Provera, or even natural estrogens and progesterone, are not conclusive when it comes to the level of protection they can provide against heart disease. All things considered, the use of natural estrogen and progesterone would be the safer choice without the potential side effects. If lowering "bad" cholesterol and raising "good" cholesterol is proven to lower the risk of heart disease, natural hormones can provide an even better level of protection than synthetic HRT.

However, reducing your risk for heart disease is more complicated than taking a pill. You must also eat a healthy diet and exercise. By changing your diet, you can go a long way toward lowering your cholesterol. Any woman at risk for heart disease should begin an exercise program (in consultation with her doctor) that includes strength training and a cardiovascular workout. If you are at great risk for heart disease, you should be getting advice from a heart specialist, not your gynecologist or internist. Don't be lulled into thinking that taking hormones—any hormone—will "vaccinate" you against heart disease.

I'm taking Provera along with Premarin to protect against endometrial cancer. Will it?

Provera was originally added to what was the standard hormone replacement regimen in 1977 to protect women against endometrial cancer. Before that, women were given Premarin alone. Then, in 1975, an article in the *New England Journal of Medicine* reported that among female patients at Kaiser Permanente medical center in San Francisco, 57 percent with endometrial cancer had used Premarin, as opposed to only 15 percent of the controls. Once this link between Premarin and endometrial cancer had been established, there was great pressure to find a drug that would offset the carcinogenic effect of Premarin. That drug was Provera, a synthetic progestin that had originally been designed for use in birth control pills. In 1977, doctors began prescribing it for use with Premarin.

Most endometrial cancer is caused by too much unopposed estrogen. Natural progesterone and synthetic progestin both oppose estrogen and thus protect women against endometrial cancer. But Provera has multiple side effects and can interfere with your body's own production of progesterone. Natural progesterone has none of these downsides and has many other benefits to your well-being (see Chapter 5, pages 74–77), and is therefore a superior choice.

I've had breast cancer. What can I do for menopausal symptoms?

It is understandable that a woman who has had breast cancer would want to approach any treatment with caution. Many doctors prescribe progesterone cream to control symptoms. Young women on tamoxifen frequently begin to experience menopausal symptoms—and here again, progesterone cream is a good choice. Also see Chapter 5, page 73, regarding estriol; there is some evidence that estriol may protect against breast cancer, and should be used in conjunction with progesterone. Another alternative is Remifemin, an herbal supplement based on black cohosh, which has been extensively tested, is safe for use by breast cancer survivors, and can help reduce or eliminate menopausal symptoms. Of course, before taking any over-the-counter product, consult with your doctor(s), including your oncologist.

Do women in menopause need to supplement testosterone?

Testosterone is an androgen hormone, meaning that it is produced in both men and women. Women, of course, produce far less of it—only about 5 percent of the testosterone a man produces. Nevertheless, testosterone is important for women. It affects your libido, helps your body recover from physical stresses, gives you energy, builds and maintains bone and muscle, and promotes a sense of well-being.

During menopause, testosterone levels can drop 50 percent. As a result, a woman can experience a loss of sexual desire; joint pain; irritability; depression; weight loss; thin, dry skin; and other problems. Conversely, too much testosterone can result in feelings of aggression, anxiety, growth of facial hair, and acne.

Women in menopause who have used testosterone replacement often report a renewed sense of vitality and increased libido. Their claims are supported by a study presented in 1998 to the North American Menopause Society by Dr. Peter Collins of the Royal Brompton Hospital in London. Sixteen postmenopausal women who were given methyltestosterone over an eighteen-month period reported an improvement in overall emotional well-being.

As with all hormone replacement, it's essential that you test your levels first and take only the amount of testosterone you need to get your hormones in proper balance. Because testosterone levels fluctuate throughout the day—they are usually higher in the morning than the afternoon—you must be careful when and how you test. Before you get tested, read Chapters 2 and 4, pages 19 and 37, and make sure the clinician understands about the time factor. If you are using a saliva test at home, follow the directions I give in Chapter 2. Should you find that you do want to replace testosterone, you'll need a prescription from your doctor; a compounding pharmacy can supply you with the natural version, not methyltestosterone, which I don't recommend. Some practitioners claim that because testosterone can convert to estrogen in the body it is safer to use the synthetic, which doesn't convert to estrogen. However, natural testosterone does not convert to estrogen automatically, but only to fill a necessary need. When you use testosterone, monitor your levels with blood tests every six months; you can reduce your dosage over time as your symptoms stabilize.

A friend in menopause is taking only progesterone to control her symptoms. She says her doctor told her she doesn't need estrogen. Can I do this too?

If your symptoms are mild, the answer may very well be yes. Many women have found that the use of progesterone—the preferred form would be a cream—can control their symptoms. As a precursor hormone (see Chapter 5, page 61), progesterone will balance your estrogen and can convert to estrogen as needed over time.

I see DHEA advertised in magazines for "mature" readers. What is it? Should I take it?

DHEA, one of the principal sex steroid hormones, has piqued the interest of the medical community in recent years. It's become a darling of some health care companies and is heavily promoted in magazines and health food stores. One of the primary reasons for this intense interest are studies that show a correlation between a drop in DHEA and increased risk of breast cancer, heart disease, Parkinson's disease, diabetes, and high blood pressure, among other ailments. But a *correlation* simply means that two things relate to each other in a way not expected on the basis of chance alone. It does not mean that low DHEA *causes* any specific condition, or that taking DHEA will prevent it.

There is no doubt that DHEA plays an extremely important role in the body. It fights disease, builds and repairs protein tissues, and is instrumental during pregnancy. The body produces more DHEA than any other sex hormone, but we are a long way from fully understanding all its functions. In both men and women, DHEA levels peak at around age 20. By the time a woman is in her sixties or seventies, her DHEA is only about 20 percent of what it was when she was young, which is probably why the idea of supplementing it seems so attractive.

Recent research suggests that in men, DHEA may someday be helpful in treating Alzheimer's disease, memory problems, chronic fatigue, obesity, and other conditions. However, the research has been done *on men only*. The field of medicine has an unfortunate history of studying men and applying the results to women. With a sex steroid hormone like DHEA, this is especially problematic.

Women who have high levels of DHEA sometimes suffer from male-pattern hair loss, facial hair growth, abdominal obesity, and other conditions. Meanwhile, the supposed positive benefits of DHEA for women, such as prevention of breast cancer, have not been established.

More worrisome is the possibility that taking DHEA—which is readily available in health food stores—may lead to endometrial cancer in women and prostate cancer in men because our bodies convert DHEA into estrogen and testosterone. Richard Sprott of the National Institute on Aging is reminded of what happened when women first used estrogen in HRT: "We saw an upswing in endometrial cancer cases until we learned to combine estrogen with progesterone. We don't know what the case is with DHEA."

In years to come, we will probably understand much more about how DHEA works, but for the time being its benefits to the average woman are outweighed by its risks. There is one exception: Women who have undergone hysterectomies and therefore are in surgical menopause may want to replace DHEA along with testosterone, estrogen, and progesterone to reconstruct a balanced hormone profile. The dose will depend upon your hormone levels. Getting the advice of a physician who is knowledgeable about hormones is invaluable for women who have had hysterectomies. Call the Natural Woman Institute (see the Resources section) for a referral if you cannot find a doctor on your own.

I hate the idea that I'm still bleeding at age 58 while taking Premarin/Provera. Will the same be true on naturals?

No. On an estrogen/progesterone regime, you may experience some spotting for the first few weeks, but then it will subside. This is one of the many positive benefits of natural hormone replacement.

Chapter Eleven

HYSTERECTOMIES AND NATURAL HORMONES

*F*ar too many women have hysterectomies unnecessarily. If you have not yet undergone surgery, I urge you to do more research and get a second opinion! If, like me, you've already had the operation, take heart. The proper combinations of natural hormones can restore your well-being, whether your hysterectomy took place decades ago or just last month.

I've had a complete hysterectomy. My doctor has prescribed estrogen, but do I also need to take progesterone?

Until recently, the conventional wisdom has been that women without a uterus do not need to include progesterone as part of their HRT because they are not at risk for endometrial (uterine) cancer. Women who have had hysterectomies, therefore, are usually given Premarin but not Provera. The Premarin/Provera protocol came into use in the 1970s, when women on high-dosage Premarin showed increased evidence of endometrial cancer. Women who'd had hysterectomies, it was reasoned, needed only to take Premarin.

This approach, which treats progesterone as merely a Band-Aid solution with no uses other than to protect against endometrial cancer, fails to take into account the extremely important role progesterone plays in balancing estrogen, building bone, and protecting against other cancers. While it's true that if you've had a hysterectomy you don't need it to safeguard against endometrial cancer, taking natural progesterone (along with a natural estrogen product) can limit water retention and weight gain, enhance the functions of your central nervous system, help balance the other hormones in your body, and potentially protect against breast cancer.

After years of taking Premarin alone, many women report multiple side effects, including weight gain, headaches, gastrointestinal problems, and lack of libido. A growing number of M.D.'s, nurse practitioners, and other health practitioners are beginning to see the value of progesterone for women who have had hysterectomies. Usually these women feel a greater sense of well-being once they begin taking progesterone, and many report a return to a feeling of normality.

If you've had a complete hysterectomy, get a full steroid panel of tests to see where your hormone levels are now (see the section in Chapter 2 titled "How to Get the Tests You Need," page 22). Also, consider replacing testosterone and perhaps DHEA.

I've had a hysterectomy but my ovaries are still intact. How do they affect my hormones? Do I need hormone replacement?

Although your ovaries are still intact, they are probably not producing enough hormones to maintain a healthy hormonal balance. In the standard hysterectomy, the branch of the uterine artery that supplies blood to the ovaries is cut and tied off. Without an adequate blood supply, the ovaries stop producing hormones properly. In cases where they do produce some, it's usually only a matter of time—three or four years—before hormone production halts altogether.

Whether you've had a complete hysterectomy or one in which your ovaries were spared, you must get a full steroid panel of tests to measure the levels of all your hormones: estrogen, progesterone, testosterone, and DHEA. When you get the results, you and your doctor can make decisions about hormone replenishment.

My doctor tells me that after my hysterectomy I will be in
"surgical menopause." How is this different from regular
menopause?

First, before having surgery, you should get a second opinion
to confirm the actual need for your hysterectomy. And don't just
rely on doctors; educate yourself before you take this serious, ir-
revocable step. Dr. Stanley West, author of *The Hysterectomy
Hoax,* believes that unless you have cancer, you probably should
not have your uterus and/or ovaries removed. Each year 600,000
hysterectomies are performed; by Dr. West's criteria, more than
500,000 of them may be unnecessary. Before you get a hysterectomy I urge you to read his book or another fine book on the
subject, *No More Hysterectomies,* by Vicki Hufnagel, M.D.

The most obvious way in which surgical menopause differs
from regular menopause is that it occurs suddenly. Normally, a
woman goes through perimenopause (which in some cases can last
ten years) and gradually reaches a time when her periods stop
altogether. Although symptoms can be unpleasant, at least they
don't hit her all at once, overnight. She has some time to adjust.
In the case of surgical menopause, there is no period of adjustment.
One day your ovaries are pumping out hormones, the next day
they're gone. If your ovaries are intact they may still produce small
amounts of hormones, but the levels usually fall short of the output prior to the hysterectomy.

Your age and how old you are when you've had your hysterectomy is also a factor. If you are in your twenties or thirties—and it
is sad indeed to have this operation so young—you may not experience symptoms until closer to menopausal age, but they may then
come with a vengeance. If you are closer to average menopausal
age, you are more likely to have symptoms immediately.

In addition to hot flashes and night sweats, symptoms of surgical menopause that may follow the operation include hair loss,
headaches, heart palpitations, fatigue, mood swings, urinary tract

problems, vaginal dryness, and loss of libido. Forty percent of hysterectomized women report becoming severely depressed after the operation, and many others no doubt suffer in silence.

In all likelihood you will need to replenish hormones after your hysterectomy. Your best defense against the symptoms of surgical menopause is a good offense. Several weeks before the procedure, do the following:

* Read up on natural hormones.

* Tell your doctor you want to use natural hormones, not synthetics. Discuss your options with him or her.

* Get your hormone levels tested prior to the operation so you have a baseline for comparison.

If your doctor or HMO is resistant to these plans, or if your doctor tells you that Premarin is his or her treatment of choice, see another doctor for advice about natural hormone replacement. Your insurance company may not pay for this visit, but even if you have to foot the bill yourself, it's well worth it.

A year ago I had a hysterectomy and was prescribed Premarin. I've already gained twenty-five pounds and can't exercise it off. Why?

The extreme weight gain suffered by some women who are given Premarin after a hysterectomy is due to too much unopposed estrogen in the system. Prior to the hysterectomy, your estrogen was being balanced, or opposed, by progesterone. Progesterone cancels out some of the properties of estrogen that lead to water retention and weight gain.

When a woman is given Premarin after her hysterectomy without having her hormone levels tested, which is the most common procedure, a number of things can go wrong. First, the "one size fits all" dose of estrogen in Premarin may be way too much for her system. In addition, her progesterone levels have also diminished as a result of the operation and so there is less available to balance the estrogen. Women do produce estrogen in parts of their body other than the ovaries—for instance, in their fat cells. If you were of average weight or heavier before the hysterectomy, by taking Premarin you may be overloading your system with estrogen.

Second, it has been standard practice for many years for doctors to prescribe estrogen but not progesterone to hysterectomized women. This is because progesterone (in the form of synthetic progestin) was originally added to HRT in order to protect women from endometrial cancer; it was thought that women without a uterus didn't need the protection of progesterone. However, progesterone performs a great many functions in the body beyond protecting against cancer. For example, it balances the properties of estrogen, as mentioned previously. Without your ovaries, or with your ovaries producing only tiny amounts of progesterone, your system may be overwhelmed by estrogen.

Both Premarin and too much natural estrogen can cause weight gain and bloating. You will not be able to diet or exercise this weight off, although you may be able to make a small dent in it. The best solution is to switch to natural hormones and, above all, get your hormone levels tested. Besides replacing estrogen and progesterone, you may want to add in testosterone. Testosterone can provide many benefits, including increased energy, bone strength, and, not least of all, improved sexual desire, something that disappears for many women after a hysterectomy.

I'm 70 and just had a hysterectomy. Do I need to replace hormones?

Although you went through the change of life years ago, there are good reasons to consider natural hormones after your hysterectomy. You're probably wondering if having your uterus, ovaries, or both removed at this stage could possibly affect your hormone levels. The answer is yes. Your ovaries continue to produce testosterone even after menopause. Low testosterone has been linked to a number of unpleasant symptoms including joint pain; irritability; depression; weight loss; thin, dry skin; and low libido. If tests show that your testosterone is low, replacing it with natural testosterone might be a prudent move. Bear in mind that even if your ovaries are left intact, their testosterone production might slow down after the hysterectomy. According to Dr. John Lee, "Even in cases in which the ovaries appear to be saved, they often quit functioning in two to three years."

There are other reasons to investigate natural hormones at this stage of your life, whether you've had a hysterectomy or not. Natural hormones have been shown to protect against Alzheimer's disease, osteoporosis, heart disease, stroke, and some types of cancer. After your hysterectomy, why not get tested for hormone levels and bone mineral density? At the very least, testing will give you a score sheet on your body's aging process. Once you're armed with the data, you and your physician can decide whether you need natural hormones.

Since my hysterectomy I have no interest in sex. Will natural hormones help?

Thousands of women have discovered, to their tremendous relief, that taking natural hormones restores their libido and sense of well-being after a hysterectomy. This is true for women who've had only their uterus removed as well as those who have had a complete hysterectomy—removal of the uterus and the ovaries.

The standard protocol after a hysterectomy is to put a woman on Premarin or a similar hormone. Very often, this not only results in unwanted side effects, but does nothing to improve her libido. We are now learning that progesterone, testosterone, and possibly

DHEA affect sex drive, so taking estrogen alone—either synthetic or natural—may not be sufficient to feel sexy again. More and more doctors are prescribing low doses of testosterone, in addition to estrogen and progesterone, to improve libido.

If you didn't get a full steroid panel of tests after your hysterectomy, do so now. With those results in hand, your doctor can write you a prescription for natural hormones that will improve your libido. You may need anywhere from one to all four hormones. If you opt for a single product, order only enough for one or two months at a time—especially at first, when your doctor will be fine-tuning the prescription.

Keep in mind that even if you still have your ovaries, they may not be producing nearly as many hormones as they did prior to the hysterectomy. You need to get tested to find out where you stand. The production of estrogen and other hormones from your ovaries may vary, and in some cases taper off altogether, over the next few years. If you get your hormones tested when things begin to feel "off," you can have your doctor readjust your prescription so that it evolves along with your changing hormone levels.

Chapter Twelve

HEALTHY BONES AND NATURAL HORMONES

*O*steoporosis was an obscure medical term until about ten years ago. Now it is on everyone's mind, especially if you're a woman over 45. Keeping your bones strong and healthy and thereby avoiding the diminished quality of life that broken bones and joint pain can bring is the key to a vital later part of life. But it's important to know what the best treatment is for you and how to avoid risky drugs that can have some benefits but also many risk factors.

I've just had a bone mineral density test and it says I'm at high risk for osteoporosis. What does that mean?

The bone mineral density (BMD) test gauges the rate at which your bones are losing their mass, or density. A woman's bone mass is at its peak when she is between 25 and 35. After that, her bone mass starts to drop at a rate of about 1 percent a year. When she reaches menopause, the annual rate of loss accelerates to 2 to 5 percent for anywhere from three to ten years; from that point on, it slows again to 1 to 1.5 percent a year.

Once you've been informed that you are at risk for osteoporosis, you must take action. If you do not, it is virtually assured that your bone mass will continue to diminish. This does not mean, however, that you necessarily have to resort to osteoporosis drugs such as Fosamax. Fortunately, by beginning a strength training regime, changing your diet, and taking natural hormone replacements and vitamin and mineral supplements, you can stop or slow the loss of bone density and even grow new bone.

Why do bones lose their mass?

Bones lose mass because of the way they grow. Two cell types are involved in the formation of bone: *osteoclasts* and *osteoblasts*. Osteoclast cells are responsible for locating old bone and dissolving it. Osteoblast cells fill the empty spaces with new bone. This process is called *remodeling*.

Like so many processes in the body, bone remodeling is a balancing act. When you're growing up, there are more osteoblasts, so your bones grow larger. After puberty, when you've reached your full height, the production of osteoblasts slows until they are in balance with the osteoclasts. After your mid-thirties, the production of osteoblasts slows down again. The osteoclasts keep removing old bone, but there aren't enough osteoblasts to replace all the empty spaces. As a result, your bones have less mass. When your bone mass is diminished past a certain point, your bones become light, brittle, and prone to fractures. This condition is osteoporosis.

Which naturals should I take for osteoporosis?

Both natural estrogens and Premarin have been shown to slow bone loss in women. There have been many studies to support this finding, but they also reveal that estrogen does not cause new bone to grow. Therefore, taking estrogen can retard osteoporosis but cannot cure it. In fact, studies using Premarin as the estrogen replacement drug have shown that it was effective for slowing bone loss for about six years into menopause. Other studies compared the rate of bone loss in women who had never taken Premarin to that of women who had taken it but given it up four years earlier. There was no discernible difference in their bone mineral density.

Somewhere along the line, the benefits of this estrogen replacement had vanished.

There is good news, however, for women who hope to maintain their bone mass and even build new bone. Groundbreaking studies by Dr. Jerilynn Prior of the University of British Columbia have shown that progesterone not only slows bone loss, but can also create new bone formation. Progesterone has no known side effects, except as related to dose (too much can cause sleepiness, for example), and it doesn't raise the risk of breast cancer, as some estrogens (especially estradiol) can if taken alone.

Studies are currently underway regarding the roles of testosterone and DHEA in building bone. Testosterone has been shown to have bone-building properties in both men and women. Researchers have found that women of all ages who have osteoporosis have lower-than-average levels of DHEA. These provocative findings may lead to reliable treatments for osteoporosis in the future.

Synthetic progesterone—progestins such as Provera—have some of the same effects on bone as natural progesterone. However, progestins have serious side effects. Stick with natural progesterone.

My friend, who is 70, is taking Evista for her osteoporosis. She says it's a designer estrogen. What does that mean?

Designer estrogens are synthetic hormones intended to protect a woman's heart and bones without the risk of uterine and breast cancer associated with standard HRT (for example, Premarin/ Provera). Designer estrogens are also known as SERMs (selective estrogen receptor modulators). Evista is the brand name for raloxifene, the first designer estrogen to receive FDA approval.

Raloxifene is now being prescribed to women with osteoporosis because in a 1997 study sponsored by raloxifene's manufacturer, Eli Lilly, the drug was found to slightly increase bone density. Specifically, women who took a daily dose of 150 milligrams had an increase of a little more than 1 percent in bone density in the lumbar spine and hip. Women taking a placebo *lost* that amount. However, the study did not look at fracture rates, which is the main issue. Raloxifene also lowered total blood cholesterol by 6.4 percent; it reduced "bad" cholesterol levels by 10 percent but did not raise "good" cholesterol levels. The study did not measure rates of heart attack or stroke, so there is no evidence that raloxifene lowers the risks for either of these.

The research showed that raloxifene does not pose the risks of breast or endometrial cancer that estrogen does, but the study had only a two-year follow-up. The very newness of raloxifene should give women pause. When doctors prescribe an estrogen drug or Fosamax to combat osteoporosis, they typically tell women to take it indefinitely, and it's likely they will give the same instructions with raloxifene. Yet we don't know how the drug will affect a woman's body five or ten years down the line, or whether its bone-saving properties will still be viable then. As with so many synthetic hormones, women must weigh the benefits with the risks. Natural progesterone can provide similar bone-creating benefits. With its record for safety, natural progesterone is a better choice.

My doctor has prescribed Fosamax for my osteoporosis. What is it?

In 1994 the drug Fosamax was introduced as a means of increasing bone mass in women with osteoporosis. Fosamax creates new bone, but it is not identical to normal human bone. For one thing, it's more brittle. And unlike normal bone, which continuously *remodels* itself (the process whereby old bone dissolves and is replaced with new bone), bone created with Fosamax is permanent. The impact this will have on a bone's ability to heal itself is still unclear.

There have been no long-term studies on Fosamax, which should instantly cause concern. Since the makers of Fosamax recommend that women use it for life, the lack of long-term studies essentially means that you will be taking it on an experimental basis.

If all this isn't enough to persuade you to stay away from this drug, a 1996 study in the *New England Journal of Medicine* reported that, if taken incorrectly, Fosamax can severely damage a woman's esophagus. The makers of Fosamax advise women to remain standing or sitting—not to lie down—for at least half an hour after ingesting the drug.

Question your doctor closely if he or she suggests using Fosamax. As of this writing, I see no reason for any woman to put herself at risk with this product. There are other, safer ways to save your bones.

Can I just take Tums with calcium for my bones?

The calcium in antacids is not easily absorbed, so it is not a good idea to rely on antacids as a source of calcium. It's much more beneficial to get your calcium through the foods you eat. For prevention of osteoporosis, your total intake of calcium should be between 800 and 1,000 milligrams daily; you can take a calcium supplement of about 300 milligrams if you like, but the rest should come from food.

Second, there are additives in antacids such as aluminum, silicone, dyes, and preservatives. While these probably won't hurt you if you take antacids every once in a while, there's no good reason to ingest them every day.

Finally, calcium alone is not enough to build healthy bones anyway. No pill alone will do the trick—especially not an antacid. In fact, calcium can't be properly incorporated into bone without a sufficient supply of magnesium and vitamin B-6. See Chapter 3 for the diet, exercise, and supplements that are most likely to give you strong, healthy bones.

Can I just exercise and improve my diet to increase bone mass?

For many women, the answer is yes. All women start losing bone mass at around age 35. If you begin strength (weight) training and eating a healthy diet at that time, you might be able to preserve strong bones without ever needing hormone replacement to stop or reverse bone loss. Even if you're 45, 55, or older, there's a possibility that exercise and diet alone will be sufficient to maintain strong bones. It all depends on how much mass you've lost. To find that out, you must take a bone mineral density test.

Strength training is essential to maintaining bone mass. Cycling, swimming, or playing tennis will not do the trick. Lifting weights or working on weight machines puts a demand on your bones that forces them to grow stronger. Other types of exercise might be wonderful for cardiovascular health, but only strength training can rebuild bone.

Eating a diet rich in calcium is good for your bones, but without weight training it won't rebuild bone mass. You should also make sure you get enough magnesium, manganese, boron, and vitamins D and K. These vitamins and minerals ensure that calcium is optimally absorbed in your body. Your diet should also include a wide variety of vegetables, which are rich in phytohormones. Just this one improvement in your diet can provide significant benefit to your bones.

If your bone mineral density test reveals substantial loss of bone mass, natural progesterone combined with diet, supplements, and strength training can often reverse the problem.

LOOKING FORWARD

There is no question that this is a very exciting time to be a woman—there is so much more freedom, so many more options and opportunities than there were for our mothers and grandmothers. But if you're happily moving up a career path, the last thing you want is to get sideswiped by monthly PMS or some gynecological mishap. Likewise, if you've just given birth, you don't want postpartum depression to deprive you of a joyful experience with your child. And a woman today does not have the option to just hide in her bedroom for a year to wait out the worst symptoms of menopause.

Many women take a certain amount of gynecological problems for granted. They think it's a price they have to pay for being a woman. Not so. As the ample evidence in this book shows, exercising and eating right, then keeping your hormones balanced—with natural hormones if necessary—will keep you healthy, fit, vibrant, and in the gynecologist's office only for regular checkups. This self-care can keep you away from unnecessary gynecological procedures that can then cascade into decades of chronic ill health.

Ignoring your body—thinking it will just somehow take care of itself or putting your health care completely in the hands of others—can have serious consequences. Over the last ten years, women have been targeted as a major market by drug companies. There has been an explosion of women's health products, including a wide variety of herbal products. A woman can be overwhelmed with choices, which is all the more reason to get a grasp of the underlying principles of how your hormones work. There are definitely many beneficial new products, many of which I recommend in this book, but there are also unnecessary or even harmful products designed to do nothing more than part you from your money. With a solid understanding of how your body works and what it needs, no matter what new products appear, you'll be prepared to evaluate them and sort out the good from the bad, the unnecessary, or the ineffectual.

My own serious illness ultimately had many blessings for me. Because my problems were so extreme, I was forced to research and dig more deeply on my own than the average woman with just hot flashes and other common problems of hysterectomy or menopause might do. Through my research, I got the added benefit of a grounding in the fundamentals of how hormones work in the body. Unfortunately, when you research deeply, you find out just how *unscientific* a lot of what passes for science actually is. This is particularly true when it comes to the dispensing of hormone replacement drugs. I learned how much of "standard HRT practice" evolved piecemeal without rigorous justification—or it was just what drug companies wanted to sell you, without enough concern for side effects. Drug companies may be willing to accept the side effects that come with their drugs, but *why should you* if you don't have to? Most side effects of standard hormone replacement drugs can be avoided by using natural hormones. The truth is that more women than you would ever want to count have suffered unnecessarily from taking the standard HRT drugs of the last forty years.

Once I recovered my health, the greatest blessing of all was feeling so well-prepared to keep myself healthy, fit, and vital for years to come. I am not often confused by conflicting information sent out through the media. I feel on top of the issues and able to read between the lines of new announcements promising "cures."

And I also feel I can take advantage of what's new and good with a more reasoned approach.

The best way to deal with anxiety and uncertainty is to educate yourself. Get away from the principle of being taken care of by others. Learn to take care of yourself. Then share your knowledge with other women. Nothing can turn around the present state of women's health care for the better than a woman-to-woman network. As I say to every woman who calls the Natural Woman Institute, *spread the word*.

RESOURCES

DOCTOR REFERRALS

The Natural Woman Institute, founded by Christine Conrad, has a nationwide database of M.D.'s and other practitioners who prescribe natural hormones. To date, we have given thousands of referrals.

Natural Woman Institute
8539 Sunset Blvd., #135
Los Angeles, CA 90069
888-489-6626
www.naturalwoman.org
E-mail: *info@naturalwoman.org*

OTHER REFERRAL RESOURCES

American College for Advancement in Medicine
P.O. Box 3427
Laguna Hills, CA 92654
800-532-3688
www.acam.org
E-mail: *acam@acam.org*

American Association of Naturopathic Physicians
601 Valley St., Suite 105
Seattle, WA 98109
206-298-0126
www.naturopathic.org/welcome.html

HealthWorld Online
www.healthy.net

RESOURCES FOR HORMONE TESTING

SALIVA HORMONE TESTING

Aeron Life Cycles
1933 Davis St., Suite 310
San Leandro, CA 94577
800-631-7900
www.aeron.com

Great Smokies Diagnostic Laboratory
63 Zillicoa St.
Asheville, NC 28801
800-522-4762 (doctors)
888-891-3061 (consumers)
www.gsdl.com

ZRT Laboratory
12505 N.W. Cornell Rd.
Portland, OR 97213
David Zava, Ph.D.
503-469-0741
E-mail: *dtzava@aol.com*

24-HOUR URINE TESTING

Meridien Valley Clinical Laboratory
Kent, WA 98042
800-234-6285

DIGESTIVE TESTS

Great Smokies Diagnostic Laboratory
(see listing on page 166)
The best resource available for a wide range of digestive
tests.

VITAMIN DEFICIENCY TESTS

SpectraCell Laboratories, Inc.
7051 Port West, Suite 100
Houston, TX 77024
800-227-5227
www.spectracell.com
E-mail: *spec1@spectracell.com*
Blood tests that measure the biochemical intracellular function of
essential micronutrients. Can help you decide on a nutritional
supplement plan.

RECOMMENDED PRODUCTS

Rx Vitamins
200 Myrtle Blvd.
Larchmont, NY 10538
800-792-2222
www.rxvitamins.com
Excellent product line distributed through doctors only.
CDA-21 is a highly recommended probiotic.

Enzymatic Therapy
825 Challenger Dr.
Green Bay, WI 54311
800-783-2286
www.enzy.com
Also distributed as PhytoPharmica. Complete vitamin,
mineral, and herbal supplement line. Distributes the
nutritional supplement Remifemin for PMS and menopause.

PhytoPharmica
800-553-2370 (doctors only)

Tyler Encapsulations
800-869-9705 (doctors only)

Prevail
2204 N.W. Birdsdale
Gresham, OR 97030
800-248-0885
www.prevail.com
E-mail: *info@prevail.com*

Vitanica
P.O. Box 1285
Sherwood, OR 97140
800-572-4712
www.vitanica.com
E-mail: *vitanica@aol.com*

Novogen
www.novogen.com
Maker of Promensil, which is available in most retail
drugstores; you can also order it directly online at
Novogen's Web site. Rimostil will be available in the fall of
2000.

COMPOUNDING PHARMACIES

The number of compounding pharmacies that work with natural hormones is growing exponentially. Just in the last year, I have discovered fifty more around the country. Don't be surprised if there is a compounder in your city that we haven't listed. Several pharmacies have large mail-order businesses and will ship anywhere in the country. They will also provide literature on natural hormones. In addition to the Natural Woman Institute, these pharmacies can often provide a doctor referral in your area.

ORGANIZATIONS

International Academy of Compounding Pharmacists (IACP)
P.O. Box 1365
Sugar Land, TX 77487
800-927-4227
Fax: 281-495-0602
www.iacprx.org
Robert Harshbarger, R.Ph., President
Over 1,000 members in the United States, Canada, and Australia. This organization will provide the name of a compounding pharmacy in your city.

National Association of Compounding Pharmacies (NACP)
4015 River Rd.
Amarillo, TX 79108
800-687-7850
Fax: 800-687-8902

Professional Compounding Centers of America, Inc. (PCCA)
9901 S. Wilcrest
Houston, TX 77099
800-331-2498
www.thecompounders.com

PHARMACIES

Canada
Northmount Pharmacy
145 East 13th St.
North Vancouver, BC V7L 2L4
800-816-5533
604-985-8241
www.northmountpharmacy.com

Pickering Village Pharmacy
59 Old Kingston Road
Ajax, ON L1T 3A5
905-683-9271

Hunter's Pharmacy
3019 Tecumseh Rd.
East Windsor, ON N8W 1G8
519-945-4333

Smith's Pharmacy
3463 Yonge St.
Toronto, ON M4N 2N3
800-361-6624 (Canada only)
416-488-2600
E-mail: *service@pharmacy.com*

Saskatoon Medical Arts Pharmacy Compounding Centre
133-750 Spadina Crescent East
Saskatoon, SK S7K 3H3
306-652-5252
at.saskyellowpages.com/medicalartspharmacy/

United States (Nationwide)
Bryce Rx Laboratories
5 Skyline Dr.
Hawthorne, NY 10531
800-798-7279
914-345-2000

Medicine Shoppe Pharmacy
800-325-1397
www.medshoppe.com
1,200 locations across the United States.

Alabama
Wellness Health & Pharmacy
2800 S. 18th St.
Birmingham, AL 35209
800-227-2627
205-879-6551

Alaska
North Pole Prescription Laboratory
167 Santa Claus Ln.
North Pole, AK 99705
907-488-8555

Arizona
Mountain View Pharmacy
10565 N. Tatum Blvd., Suite B118
Paradise Valley, AZ 85253
480-948-7065

Cactus Professional Pharmacy & Compounding Center
4045 E. Bell Rd., Suite 101
Phoenix, AZ 85032
602-971-6950

Apothecary Shop of Scottsdale
10250 N. 92nd St., Suite 105
Scottsdale, AZ 85258
888-276-8353
602-451-3771
www.theapothecaryshop.com
E-mail: *jmusil@syspac.com*

Women's International Pharmacy
13925 W. Meeker Blvd., Suite 13
Sun City West, AZ 85375
800-279-5708
623-214-7700
www.wipws.com
E-mail: *info@wipws.com*

Reed's Compounding Pharmacy
2729 E. Speedway Blvd.
Tucson, AZ 85716
520-318-4421

Arkansas
Lee Pharmacy
4300 Grand Ave.
Fort Smith, AR 72904
800-209-9940
501-782-8689
www.leepharmacy.com

California
B&B Pharmacy
10244 Rosecrans Ave.
Bellflower, CA 90706
800-231-8905

Compounding Pharmacy of Beverly Hills
9629 W. Olympic Blvd.
Beverly Hills, CA 90212
310-284-8675

Triad Compounding
11090 E. Artesia Blvd., Suite H
Cerritos, CA 90703
800-851-7900
562-468-4311

Steven's Pharmacy, A Harbor Drug Company Pharmacy
1525 Mesa Verde Dr.
East Costa Mesa, CA 92626
800-352-3784
714-540-8911
www.stevensrx.com

Valley Drug and Compounding
16928 Ventura Blvd.
Encino, CA 91316
877-482-6231
818-788-0635
www.1pharmacy.com
E-mail: *info@1pharmacy.com*

Medical-Dental Pharmacy
6327 N. Fresno, #104
Fresno, CA 93710
800-794-2832
559-439-1190
www.rxcompounders.com
E-mail: *mdpii@aol.com*

University Compounding Pharmacy
P.O. Box 953
Imperial Beach, CA 91933
www.ucprx.com
E-mail: *ucp@ucprx.com*

Park Pharmacy and Compounding Center
250 E. Yale Loop, Suite C
Irvine, CA 92604
949-551-7195
www.parkrx.com

California Pharmacy and Compounding Center
307 Placentia Ave.
Newport Beach, CA 92663
800-575-7776
949-642-8057
www.californiapharmacy.com
E-mail: *cathy@californiapharmacy.com*

Central Avenue Pharmacy
133 15th St.
Pacific Grove, CA 93950
800-501-9715
831-373-1225

Panorama Compounding Pharmacy
8215 Van Nuys Blvd.
Panorama City, CA 91402
800-247-9767
818-988-7979
www.panoramapharmacy.com
E-mail: *panorap@aol.com*

Phoenix Pharmacy
2523 E. Washington Blvd.
Pasadena, CA 91104
818-791-7600

Rohnert Park Drugs
969A Golf Course Dr.
Rohnert Park, CA 94928
800-448-4355
707-586-0788

Four-Fifty Sutter Pharmacy
450 Sutter, Suite 410
San Francisco, CA 94108
415-392-4137

Leiter's Park Avenue Pharmacy
1756 Park Ave.
San Jose, CA 95126
800-292-6773
408-292-6772
www.leiterrx.com

Santa Clara Drug—The Compounding Shop
2453 Forest Ave.
San Jose, CA 95128
800-646-2453
408-296-5015
www.scdrug.com
E-mail: *info@scdrug.com*

Airport Compounding Pharmacy
3250 Pico Blvd.
Santa Monica, CA 90405
888-450-7555
310-450-7555

Jaye Pharmacy
13322 Riverside Dr.
Sherman Oaks, CA 91423
818-789-8111

Oaks Pharmacy
4940 Van Nuys Blvd.
Sherman Oaks, CA 91403
818-990-3784

Myers Apothecary Shop
238 Hospital Dr., Suite A
Ukiah, CA 95482
707-468-8991
www.myersapothecary.com

Doc's Pharmacy & Home Health Center
112 La Casa Via, Suite 100
Walnut Creek, CA 94598
800-796-4937
925-939-6311
E-mail: *rxmixer@ix.netcom.com*

Eddie's Pharmacy
8500 Melrose Ave.
West Hollywood, CA 90069
310-358-2400

Colorado
College Pharmacy
833 N. Tejon St.
Colorado Springs, CO 80903
800-888-9358
719-634-4861

Belmar Pharmacy
12860 W. Cedar Dr., #210
Lakewood, CO 80228
800-525-9473
303-763-5533

Columbine Drugs
2295 W. Eisenhower Blvd.
Loveland, CO 80538
970-663-7100

Monument Pharmacy
115C 2nd St.
P.O. Box 511
Monument, CO 80132
800-595-7565
719-481-2209

Connecticut
Prescription Specialties
555 Highland Ave.
Cheshire, CT 06410
800-861-0933
www.rxspecialties.com
E-mail: *info@rxspecialties.com*

Arrow Prescription Center
972 Main St.
Willimantic, CT 06226
860-423-1125

Florida
Pharmacy Specialists of Central Florida
650 Maitland Ave.
Altamonte Springs, FL 32701
407-260-7022
E-mail: *spratt@aol.com*

Weise Prescription Shop
4343 Colonial
Jacksonville, FL 32210
904-338-1564

Universal Arts Pharmacy
6500 W. 4th Ave., Suite 4
Hialeah–Miami Lakes, FL 33012
305-556-2673

Thayer's Colonial Pharmacy
1101 E. Colonial Dr.
Orlando, FL 32803
800-848-4809
407-862-8084

Family Pharmacy
3644 Webber St.
Sarasota, FL 34232
941-921-6645

Kinnard's Pharmacy
2075 Siesta Dr.
Sarasota, FL 34239
800-631-2667
www.@kinnardspharmacy.com

Hoyes Natural Pharmacy
3215 S. MacDill Ave.
Tampa, FL 33629
800-788-8123
813-839-8861
E-mail: *info@hoyesnaturalpharmacy.com*

Georgia
Central Pharmacy Services
1819 Peachtree Rd. NE
Atlanta, GA 30309
404-351-8366
www.centralpharmacy.com

Concord Drugs
5555 Peachtree Dunwoody Rd., NE
Atlanta, GA 30342
404-252-3607

Christian's Pharmacy
1032 Main St.
Forest Park, GA 30297
404-366-4321

Monfort Compounding Center
105 N. Perry St.
Lawrenceville, GA 30045
888-540-2438
770-963-2813
pharmacycare.com

Trumarx Drugs
501 Gordon Ave.
Thomasville, GA 31792
800-552-9997
912-226-8700

Idaho
Medicine Man Pharmacy
1114 Ironwood Dr.
Coeur d'Alene, ID 83814
208-666-2502
www.rx2u.com

Illinois
Lincoln Medical Apothecary
157 S. Lincoln Ave.
Aurora, IL 60505
800-391-9819
630-892-7777

Schott's Pharmacy Care Center
800 W. Bluff St.
Marseilles, IL 61341
815-795-2700

Martin Avenue Pharmacy
10 W. Martin Ave.
Naperville, IL 60540
630-355-6400
www.martinavenue.com

Indiana
Hollon's Panorama Pharmacy
2517 E. 10th St.
Anderson, IN 46012
800-682-3059
765-644-8851
www.hollonspharmacies.com

Kentucky
PRN Compounders
3030 Burlew Blvd.
Owensboro, KY 42303
800-216-8699
270-685-0402
If you call the 800 number, you will be asked to enter a
PIN, which is 0929.

Louisiana
Central Drugs
125 E. Thomas St.
Hammond, LA 70401
504-345-5120
E-mail: *centraldrugs@i-55.com*

Maryland
Professional Arts Pharmacy
1101 N. Rolling Rd.
Baltimore, MD 21228
800-832-9285
410-747-6870

Edwards Pharmacy
Commerce and Water Sts.
P.O. Box 340
Centreville, MD 21617
800-310-4312
410-758-1715
www.edwardspharmacy.com

Massachusetts
Conlin's Pharmacy
30 Lawrence St.
Methuen, MA 01844
888-266-5467
978-683-4561
www.conlinsnet.com
E-mail: *SKalil98@aol.com*

Birds Hill Pharmacy
401 Great Plains Ave.
Needham, MA 02492
888-500-2660
781-449-0550

Heights Pharmacy
882 Highland Ave.
Needham Heights, MA 02494
781-444-2688

Michigan
Diplomat Pharmacy
G-3320 Beecher Rd.
Flint, MI 48532
810-732-8720
www.diplomatpharmacy.com

Quest Pharmaceuticals
2951 S. Adams Rd.
Rochester Hills, MI 48326
888-455-1248
800-455-1248

South Lyon Family Pharmacy
116 N. Lafayette
South Lyon, MI 48178
248-437-6225
www.southlyonpharmacy.com
E-mail: *pharmacy@ccainc.net*

Healthway Pharmacy
1008 N. Saginaw
P.O. Box 148
St. Charles, MI 48655
800-742-7527
517-865-9971
www.healthwayrx.com
E-mail: *michaelrph@aol.com*

Minnesota
Custom-Rx Compounding Pharmacy
6519 Nicollet Ave. South, Suite 201
Richfield, MN 55423
612-866-2211
www.customrx.com

Missouri
O'Brien Pharmacy
4321 Washington, Suite 2020
Kansas City, MO 64111
800-627-4360
816-531-6763

Miller Professional Pharmacy
228 Marshall St.
Platte City, MO 64079
816-858-2400
millerrx.fountain.net

Nebraska
Kubat Pharmacy
4924 Center St.
Omaha, NE 68106
800-782-9988
402-558-8888

Nevada
Medical Center Compounding Pharmacy
3675 S. Rainbow Blvd., #103
Las Vegas, NV 89103
800-723-7455
702-873-8455
www.mccpharmacy.com

New Hampshire
Bedford Pharmacy
101 Plaza, 209 Route 101
Bedford, NH 03110
800-662-6333
603-472-3919
www.bedfordrx.com.
E-mail: *rlpetrin@bedfordrx.com*

The Apothecary
35 Main St.
Keene, NH 03431
603-357-0200

Sullivan Drug Store
104 Main St.
P.O. Box 465
Lancaster, NH 03584
800-442-4606
603-788-2751
www.sullivandrug.com

New Jersey
Rock Ridge Pharmacy
191 Rock Rd.
P.O. Box 605
Glen Rock, NJ 07456
201-444-4190
www.rockridgerx.com

Hopewell Pharmacy and Compounding Center
1 W. Broad St.
Hopewell, NJ 08525
800-792-6670
609-466-1960

Stokes Medical Arts Pharmacy
639 Stokes Rd.
Medford, NJ 08055
800-754-5222
609-654-5222
www.stokesrx.com

Wedgewood Village Pharmacy
279 Egg Harbor Rd., #C
Sewell, NJ 08080
609-589-4200

Millers Community Pharmacy Center
678 Wyckoff Ave.
Wyckoff, NJ 07481
888-891-3334
201-891-3333
www.millershomecare.com

New York
Fallon Wellness Pharmacy
282 Grooms Rd.
Clifton Park, NY 12065
800-890-1137
518-371-5922
E-mail: *rxs4future@aol.com*

Apthorp Pharmacy
2201 Broadway
New York, NY 10024
212-877-3480

Lindsay Drug
416 5th Ave.
Troy, NY 12182
888-650-3784
518-235-2522
www.lindsaydrug.com

North Carolina
The Prescription Center
915 Hay St.
Fayetteville, NC 28305
800-682-4664
Emerg. pager: 910-307-9650
www.rxfixer.com

Tom Jones Health & Wellness Center
107 Vandora Springs Rd.
Garner, NC 27529
919-772-4737
E-mail: *tomjones@mindspring.com*

North Dakota
Dakota Pharmacy
717 E. Main Ave.
P.O. Box 835
Bismarck, ND 58501
800-290-7028
701-255-1881
www.dakotarx.com
E-mail: *sarentig@dakotarx.com*

Ohio
Ritzman Natural Health Pharmacies
800-215-5898
www.ritzmanpharmacies.com
Eight locations in Ohio.

Scarbrough Pharmacy
1809 S. Main
Findlay, OH 45840
877-267-3791
419-423-1513
www.anaturalpharmacy.com
E-mail: *info@anaturalpharmacy.com*

Oklahoma
Lassiter Discount Drug
3401 S.E. 29th St.
Del City, OK 73115
888-506-0636
405-677-0549
www.lassiterdrug.com
E-mail: *lassiter@oklahoma.net*

Innovative Pharmacy Solutions
1716 S. Kelly
Edmonds, OK 73013
800-441-8706
405-330-3619

Oregon
Broadway Apothecary
10 West 17th Ave.
Eugene, OR 97401
888-644-9382
541-684-9352

Strohecker's Pharmacy
2855-A S.W. Patton Rd.
Portland, OR 97201
503-222-4822
www.stroheckersrx.com
E-mail: *beavron@aol.com*

Pennsylvania
Lundberg Pharmacy
58 E. 4th St.
Emporium, PA 15834
888-792-6737
814-486-3310

Hazle Drugs Apothecary
20 N. Laurel St.
Hazleton, PA 18201
800-439-2026
717-454-2670
www.hazledrugs.com

Williams Apothecary
201 E. Chesnut St.
Lancaster, PA 17602
717-393-3814
E-mail: *custom@apoth.com*

Library Pharmacy & Compounding Pharmacy
P.O. Box 83
2800 Brownsville Rd.
Library, PA 15129
888-646-6016
www.librarypharmacy.com

Yakim's Compounding Pharmacy
7901 Saltsburg Rd., Suite 102
Pittsburgh, PA 15239
800-368-3112
412-793-5230
E-mail: *jyakim@aol.com*

Rhode Island
Pawtuxet Valley Prescription and Surgical Center
59 Sandy Bottom Rd.
Coventry, RI 02816
877-266-7686
401-821-0600
www.pvpsc.com
E-mail: *lrb@pvpsc.com*

Prescription Compounding Specialists of RI
1145 Reservoir Ave., Suite 202
Cranston, RI 02920
401-429-0330

South Carolina
Medifare Drug Center
300 W. Pine St.
Blacksburg, SC 29702
800-527-9217
864-839-6384

Tennessee
Clark & Palin Pharmacy
121 Bluff City Hwy.
Bristol, TN 37620
800-263-8890
423-764-4136

Lakeside Pharmacy
4632 Hwy. 58 North
Chattanooga, TN 37416
800-523-1486
423-894-3222

Delk Pharmacy
1515 Hatcher Ln.
Columbia, TN 38401
931-388-3952

Texas
Abrams Royal Pharmacy
8220 Abrams Rd.
Dallas, TX 75231
214-349-8000

Apothe'Cure
13720 Midway Rd., Suite 109
Dallas, TX 75244
800-969-6601
214-490-1618
214-960-6601

Dougherty's Pharmacy
515 Preston
Royal Village
Dallas, TX 75208
800-734-1615
214-363-4318
www.doughertys-ravens.com

Raven's Pharmacy
500 W. Jefferson
Dallas, TX 75208
800-767-9744
214-946-2155
www.doughertys-ravens.com

Med-Shop Total Care Pharmacy
800-867-6762
www.med-shop.com
Three locations in eastern Texas.

Flower Mound Pharmacy & Herbal Alternatives
1001 Cross Timbers Rd., Suite 1050
Flower Mound, TX 75028
972-355-4614
E-mail: *pharmacist@fmpharmacy.com*

Green Park Pharmacy
7515 S. Main, Suite 150
Houston, TX 77030
713-795-5812

Midway Park Pharmacy
2700 W. Pleasant Run Rd., Suite 250
Lancaster, TX 75146
972-223-2623

Baggett Pharmacy
1710 College Ave.
Levelland, TX 79336
800-540-3540
806-894-7347
www.pharmvac.com

Cap Rock Discount Drugs
2625 50th St.
Lubbock, TX 79413
806-792-2713

Rediger's Pharmacy
724 S. Eddy, Box 1760
Pecos, TX 79772
800-588-1096
915-445-4916

Pharmcare Pharmacy & Medical
2206 E. Broadway, Suite F
Pearland, TX 77581
800-883-0803
281-485-7272
www.pharmcare.net

The Wellness Store of the Pill Box Pharmacy
800-888-3360
210-614-3360
Five locations in the San Antonio Area.

Kinsey's Pharmacy
1420 WSW Loop 323
Tyler, TX 75701
903-534-5468
www.kinseyspharmacy.com

Advanced Pharmaceutical Services
807 S. Beckham Ave.
Tyler, TX 75701
800-491-0074
903-592-8283
E-Mail: *info@goodspharmacy.com*

Utah
MedQuest Pharmacy
6965 Union Park Center, Suite 100
Salt Lake City, UT 84047
888-222-2956
801-566-5350
www.medquestpharmacy.com

Virginia
Medical Center Pharmacy
10721 Main St.
Fairfax, VA 22030
800-723-7455

Washington
Bellgrove Pharmacy
1535 116th Ave. NE
Bellevue, WA 98004
800-446-2123

Poulsbo Drug Store
18911 Front St., NE
P.O. Box 38
Poulsbo, WA 98370
800-882-2029 (Washington only)
360-779-2737

Beall's Pharmacy
618 S. Meridian, Suite A
Puyallup, WA 98371
877-845-0451
253-845-8444
E-mail: *beallspharmacy@email.msn.com*

Kelley-Ross Pharmacy
1120 Harvard Ave.
Seattle, WA 98122
206-324-6990
www.kelley-rossrx.com

Kelley-Ross Pharmacy
507 Olive Way
Seattle, WA 98101
206-622-3565
www.kelley-rossrx.com

Union Avenue Pharmacy
2302 S. Union Ave.
Tacoma, WA 98405
253-752-1705

West Virginia
Colony Drug
2801 Robert C. Byrd Dr.
Beckley, WV 25801
304-252-5305
E-mail: *colony@inetone.net*

Wisconsin
Madison Pharmacy Associates
Women's Health America Group
429 Gammon Place
Madison, WI 53719
800-558-7046

Women's International Pharmacy
5708 Monona Dr.
Madison, WI 53716-3152
800-279-5708
608-221-7800
www.wipws.com
E-mail: *info@wipws.com*

Island Pharmacy Services
P.O. Box 1412
Woodruff, WI 54568
800-328-7060
www.islandpharmacy.com

BIBLIOGRAPHY

Ahlgrimm, Marla, and John Kells. *The HRT Solution*. Garden City, NY: Avery, 1999.

Albertazzi, Paola. "The Effect of Dietary Soy Supplementation on Hot Flushes." *Obstetrics and Gynecology*, January 1998.

Bachmann, Gloria. "Estrogen and Androgen Improve Variety of Symptoms in Post-Menopausal Patients." Panel discussion sponsored by the University of Medicine and Dentistry of New Jersey, July 30, 1998.

Bolton, Judy. "Byproduct of Premarin Damages DNA in a Way That Could Cause Breast Cancer." *Chemical Research and Toxicology*, January 1998.

Brody, Jane E. "Estrogen and Alzheimer's." *New York Times*, June 18, 1997.

Collins, Peter. "The Addition of Methyltestosterone to Estrogen Replacement Therapy." Study presented at the North American Menopause Society Conference 9th Annual Meeting, September 16–19, 1998, Toronto, Canada.

Crouse, John, and Gregory Burke. "Soy Component Lowers Cholesterol." Study presented at the American Heart Association's 38th Annual Conference on Cardiovascular Disease and Dysfunction, March 20, 1998.

Hanley, Jesse Lynn. Interview by Lynette Padwa, October 23, 1998.

Hufnagel, Vicki G. *No More Hysterectomies*. New York: Plume, 1989.

Laux, Marcus, and Christine Conrad. *Natural Woman, Natural Menopause.* New York: HarperCollins, 1997.

Lee, John R. *What Your Doctor May Not Tell You About Menopause.* New York: Warner Books, 1996.

——— "Preventing Breast Cancer with Progesterone." *John R. Lee, M.D. Medical Letter*, April 1998, p. 1–3.

Lee, John R., Jesse Hanley, and Virginia Hopkins. *What Your Doctor May Not Tell You About Premenopause.* New York: Warner Books, 1999.

Northrup, Christiane. Interview on HRT. *International Journal of Pharmaceutical Compounding,* January–February 1998, p. 12–17.

Physician's Desk Reference. Montvale, NJ: Medical Economics, 1999.

Schardt, David, and Stephen Schmidt. "DHEA: Not Ready for Prime Time." *Nutrition Action Healthletter,* March 1997, p. 3–5.

Schmidt, Peter. "Estrogen May Play Role in Mood Swings." *New England Journal of Medicine*, January 22, 1998.

Sears, Barry. *The Anti-Aging Zone.* New York: HarperCollins, 1999.

Shaak, Carolyn V. Interview by Lynette Padwa, Needham, Massachusetts, October 14, 1998.

"Soy Isoflavones: Can These Nutrients Help Protect Against Women's Health Problems?" *The Nutrition Reporter*, July 1997, p. 1.

Warren, Michelle. "Crinone 4% Used In Treatment of Secondary Amenorrhea in Professional Ballerinas." Study presented at symposium, "Treatment of Women with Subnormal or Absent Ovarian Function: What's New and Novel," sponsored by Wyeth-Ayerst Laboratories, New Orleans, Louisiana, May 13, 1998.

Waterhouse, Debra. *Outsmarting the Midlife Fat Cell.* New York: Hyperion, 1998.

West, Stanley. *The Hysterectomy Hoax.* New York: Main St. Books, 1994.

Wright, Jonathan V., and John Morgenthaler. *Natural Hormone Replacement.* Petaluma, CA: Smart, 1997.

Zava, David. "Don't Go Overboard with Soy Foods." Interview on HRT. *John R. Lee, M.D. Medical Letter*, May 1998, p. 5–6.

INDEX

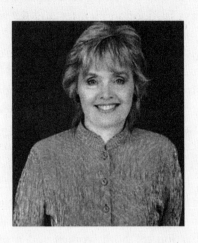

ABOUT THE AUTHOR

A Woman's Guide to Natural Hormones *follows the bestsell-ing* Natural Woman, Natural Menopause *(HarperCollins, May 1997), co-authored with Dr. Marcus Laux. Previously, Con-rad's career ranged from movies, theater, publishing, and New York City politics. She is best known for writing the original screenplay for* Junior, *the widely acclaimed movie starring Arnold Schwarzenegger, Danny DeVito, and Emma Thompson, in which Conrad takes on the issue of possible male pregnancy.*

In 1970, Conrad was appointed by then New York City Mayor John Lindsay as head of the city's Film, Television and Theatre Office. Under her direction the office shepherded such ma-jor motion pictures as *The Godfather* and *The French Connection*. After a four-year stint with Mayor Lindsay, Conrad turned to pub-lishing, first at Bantam Books, then as a Senior Editor at Warner

Books. In 1982 she began working as a screenwriter and sold numerous screenplays for motion pictures and television. For television, she wrote the #1 ABC movie, *Love Thy Neighbor*.

But along with the career success of *Junior* came serious illness, and it was during this period that she found herself searching for a "natural estrogen." After being told by her doctors that there were no alternatives to standard hormone drugs, she eventually was led to her successful treatment with natural plant-derived hormones. The difficulty she had in finding this treatment galvanized Conrad's interest in getting women the help they deserved. To further that end beyond writing the books, Conrad founded the Natural Woman Institute, a nonprofit institution dedicated to helping women find practitioners who use natural hormones; and to providing education for both women and professionals in the use of natural hormonal and nutritional therapies for women of all ages.

She can be reached at the Natural Woman Institute; *www. naturalwoman.org*; E-mail: *info@naturalwoman.org*.